# OVERCOMING ALCOHOL
# 摆脱酗酒

## 50 WAYS TO QUIT ALCOHOL OR REDUCE ITS USE
## 戒酒或减少饮酒量的 50 种方法

### T S Gill MD
### T·S·基尔博士

DEDICATED

TO

THE HIGHER POWER
献给更高层次的人类精神力量

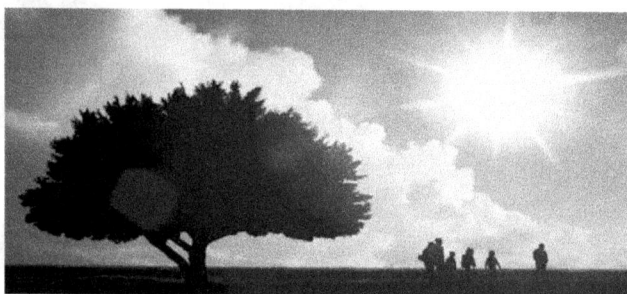

You can Do It 您可以做到

## DISCLAIMER
### 免责申明

This book is for informational purposes only. Please consult with your doctor before implementing any of the treatment strategies. The purpose of this book is to motivate you to seek help and acquaint you with the different treatment options. This is not a contract to provide medical services for alcoholism, or other conditions. The intent is to motivate you and to help you engage more fully with your doctor about your detox and rehabilitation.

本书仅作参考之用。请在实施任何治疗方案前，向医生咨询。本书的用意在于促使您寻求帮助，并对不同的治疗方法有所了解。它不是为酗酒或其他状况，提供医疗服务的一份合约，而意在促使并帮助您更充分地与医生配合，戒除酒瘾，实现康复。

## ACKNOWLEDGMENT
## 感 谢 信

I would like to acknowledge the many fine colleagues, and friends who have displayed exemplary clinical acumen and caring. I am in greater debt to individuals and their families who have shared their struggles and heartache that comes along with alcoholism in themselves or their family member. They are a testament to the ability of the human spirit to overcome challenges

我想感谢许多同事，他们医术精湛、为人谦和；我还想感谢多位朋友，他们展现了值得学习的临床观察力和护理能力；我更想感谢将自身或家庭成员与酗酒进行的抗争，以及为此而承受的痛苦与我分享的个人及其家庭成员。他们证明了人类意识能够战胜各种挑战。

You can Do It 您可以做到

# TABLE OF CONTENTS
# 目录

You can Do It 您可以做到

# ABOUT THE AUTHOR
## 作者简介

Dr. Tirath S Gill went to medical school at Govt. Medical College, Jabalpur, India and finished his residency in Psychiatry at Austin, Texas and at Yale School of Medicine in 1993. He also completed a fellowship in Chemical Dependency at Yale in 1994. He has been Board Certified by the American Board of Psychiatry and Neurology in General Psychiatry, Forensic Psychiatry, Addiction Psychiatry and Psychosomatic Medicine. He has taken several leadership positions with the Department of Veteran Affairs, and with the California Department of State Hospitals. He currently is the Chief Psychiatrist at the Substance Abuse Treatment Facility, in Corcoran, CA.

提拉特·S·基尔博士曾就读于印度贾巴尔普尔政府医科大学；并于 1993 年在美国德州奥斯丁及耶鲁医学院，完成精神病学住院实习；1994 年完成耶鲁大学药物依赖研究工作。基尔博士已经成为了美国普通精神病学、法医神经病学、成瘾精神病学及身心医学精神病学与神经学会的执业医生。此外，他还任职过退伍军人事务部部长、加州公立医院事务部部长。目前，他是加州科克伦物质滥用治疗机构的首席精神病学家。

# You can Do It 您可以做到

## PREFACE
## 前言

I had been mulling over the title of a simple book on overcoming alcohol. As I was driving to work on a highway in Central California, a Paul Simon song came on the radio with the theme that there must be 50 ways to leave your lover. If you have never heard the song or haven't heard this song in a while, you should really give it another listen.

我曾一直为命名一本简单易懂的书而绞尽脑汁，这本书与摆脱酗酒有关。当我驾车行驶在加州中部的高速公路上时，收音机里传来了保罗·西蒙的歌，歌名叫做"必定存在的离开爱人的50种方法"。如果从未听过这首歌，或者没有听完它，那么，您真的应该再听一次。

The famous songwriter had written something similar to this book's theme. Well, not exactly similar.

歌曲的作者非常有名，他写出了与本书相似的主题。当然，似也不似。

In his inimitable wisdom, he had penned a whimsical song of love and leaving. I thought it contained insights that could be applied to leaving alcohol and other addictions. In the lyrics, a kindred voice tells the silent, and we suppose perplexed man that the problem is mostly in his head.

他用无与伦比的智慧，用歌曲描绘了爱与离别的反复无常。我认为其中包含了深刻的见解，可能适用于摆脱酒瘾或其他成瘾。歌曲中，一个亲切的男声，用歌词诉说着欲语还休，让我们想到了长期承受酗酒之痛的人。

Truer words could not have been said for the alcoholic.

没有比它更真实地道出酗酒者困惑与无助的表达了。

The basis for the disease does indeed lie in the mind of the person with alcohol problems. It is in the mind that the various anxieties and urges reside. Urges that propel the continued use of alcohol despite all the negative setbacks.

事实上，酗酒的根源存在于酗酒者的意识中。各种焦虑与冲动，都存在于人的意识之中。尽管酗酒带来了种种消极萎靡、挫折不断，冲动仍然可以促使人不断酗酒。

This lovely friend in the song continues and chides the stricken man, that she does not mean to be crude, but there must be 50 ways to leave your lover. The point of this being that it is easier for him to leave his problem than he is making it out to be.

歌中，可爱的歌手继续斥责陷入病态的男人，告诉他的爱人不要让自己变得粗鲁，因为一定有 50 种方法，可以摆脱这个男人。关键在于，对这个男人而言，逃避问题比战胜问题更容易。

The truth is that it is easy to leave alcohol, once a decision has been made. To a person trapped in the toxic relationship, be it with alcohol or a person, all options seem closed, and one can develop a pessimistic and nihilistic tunnel vision about the problem of alcohol. The person caught in this fog of indecision has to be shaken up and told that there **are** "50 ways to leave".

事实上，摆脱酗酒很容易，<u>只要下定决定</u>。对于深陷这种有害关系的个人而言，与酒或酒友相伴，会让自己别无选择，还会因此而产生悲观厌世、虚无妄想的幻觉。优柔寡断的酗酒者，必须得到唤醒，并获知**现成**的 "50 种摆脱酗酒的方法。"

Getting over alcohol and leaving the dependence is easy once a decision to quit and leave alcohol behind is made.

只要做出了戒酒并远离酒精的决定，就能轻而易举地摆脱酗酒，告别对它的依赖。

This book offers the 50 or more ways to leave. The number 50 is just metaphorical, just as it is in the song.

这本书提供的戒酒方法有 50 种或更多。数字 50，不过是一种象征意义，正如那首歌中的含义一样。

Some of these ways may have been obvious; others are not so obvious to the ordinary person. The individual may have believed that the only way out is to suffer through a horrible detox and a humiliating confrontation daily by a judgmental counselor intent on beating out the last shred of self-respect.

对于普通人而言，其中的一些方法可能已司空见惯，另一些则不太常见。有人或许认为，让自己摆脱酒瘾的唯一方法，是熬过令人恐惧的脱瘾治疗，耻辱地每天面对严厉的戒酒顾问，坚决地打碎自己的最后一丝自尊。

The song says, "Just make a plan Stan and set yourself free."

那首歌唱到："斯丹，制定一个计划，让自己获得自由。"

This book also says, make a decision to quit and set yourself free. The song tells Roy not to be coy and for Jack just to slip out the back. The point of this is that you don't have to be fancy but to use whatever works. You can start small by decreasing the amount of alcohol slightly at first. The point being that there are many choices, just find what works for you. It doesn't matter what exit you choose, just quit drinking. Just break it off. And yes, there are 50 ways to leave.

本书也写到，做出决定戒酒并让自己摆脱束缚。歌曲告诫诺伊无需感到羞耻，而杰克只需要悄悄离开。这句歌词的关键，在于不要抱有幻想，而要采取任何行之有效的方法。首先，你可以减少饮酒量，迈出自己的这一小步。选择的方法多种多样，只要找到适合自己的，这才是重点。选择无关至要，只要能戒酒，让习惯戛然而止。是的，改变的方法有很多。


Once you leave, don't ever go back.

一旦抽身而出，就不要再回头。


I have found that Individuals who have recovered from alcohol dependence and other addictions are often tremendous people with high drive and a certain level of honesty. They are capable of high achievement once they attain sobriety and get help for any personal issues. The many recovered and highly successful alcoholics in all walks of life are proof that the disease of alcoholism can be overcome.

我发现，摆脱酒精依赖和其他不良嗜好而康复的人，通常具有强烈的上进心，且为人诚实。只要戒酒，获得对任何个人问题的帮助，他们就有能力取得巨大的成就。各行各业都有许多成功摆脱酗酒，实现脱瘾康复的人，他们证明了这种病是可以战胜的。


You may find some concepts repeated. This is usually to add to or to clarify a different aspect of an earlier discussion.

您可能发现了一些重复的理念。通常，重复的目的是对前面探讨的不同方面，进行补充说明或澄清。

# You can Do It 您可以做到

I hope you will be able to get some ideas that appeal to you. There are many roads to the destination of sobriety. Enjoy the book and be open to the many ways.

希望您可以从中收获一些对自己有用的观点。条条道路通罗马。玩味本书，让自己开卷有益。

T S Gill MD

T・S・基尔博士

# AN IMPORTANT WORD OF CAUTION
## 重要提示

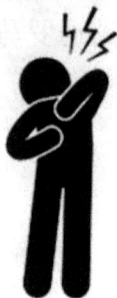

突然中止饮酒可以导致并发症—因此，不建议突然中止饮酒。

脱瘾治疗期间，应尽快开始服用硫胺素 100 毫克片剂，一日一次或两次，防止神经学并发症出现。

最好在对停止饮酒的酗酒者提供脱瘾治疗或其他能量补充前，以静脉滴注或肌注方式给药硫胺素 100 毫克。

Although a vast majority of the detoxes are safe, serious complications can occur on some occasions.

尽管绝大多数脱瘾治疗是安全的，但有时也会出现严重的并发症。

Quitting cold turkey from alcohol or in other words, suddenly stopping alcohol use if you drink daily, is not recommended. Such sudden stoppage in the context of daily alcohol use is dangerous, and there can be severe complications. The most dangerous of these is called delirium tremens or DT's. This can have a 25% mortality rate if not treated. This means one out of 4 people can die if the condition is not recognized and treated in a medical setting. The associated medical conditions can be worsened by the withdrawal related to rise in blood pressure and heart rate.

不建议酗酒者突然停止饮酒，或换言之，每日饮酒者突然停止饮酒。突然停止饮酒很危险，可以引起严重的并发症。其中，最危险的并发症称为震颤性谵妄或 DT。若不经治疗，其死亡率可达 25%。

这意味着在病症未经察觉，并以药物施治的情况下，每 4 人中有 1 人会死亡。酗酒者的身体状况，会因为突然停止饮酒所导致的血压升高和心跳加速而恶化。

Some indicators of an emerging delirium tremens are the following: confusion, hallucinations, excessive shaking or convulsions. If these occur, the individual will require admission to an emergency room for closer medical monitoring and treatment.

The other symptoms of withdrawal include the following: nausea, an increase in heart rate, a rise in blood pressure; mild shaking or tremors, headaches, sweating, and anxiety. If these are noted, it indicates that the dose of the medications used for withdrawal should be increased.

提示震颤性谵妄出现的部分指征如下：意识模糊、幻觉、过度震颤或抽搐。如出现这些症状，需将患者送入急救室，进行更密切地医疗监测与治疗。停止饮酒的其他症状包括如下：恶心、心跳加速、血压升高、轻度震颤或颤抖、头痛、出汗及焦虑。若发现这些症状，表明用于停止饮酒症状的药量应增加。

Detoxification from alcohol should be done in consultation with a doctor who is familiar with the withdrawal complications  and with  the  managing of them. This book speaks of the different ways that alcohol use can be discontinued or reduced. This is for informational purposes only and not a contract  for engagement in medical therapy. The purpose of the information is to start a conversation with your doctor. The doctor can guide you about the specifics of treatment that is right for your situation and can also provide referrals to alcohol and substance counselors, AA meetings or a detox center as needed.

进行脱瘾治疗，应咨询熟悉停止饮酒并发症，及其治疗方法的医生。本书就中断或减少饮酒的方法，进行了阐述。仅作为参考之用，不是进行药物治疗的合约。本书的用意在于帮助您开始与医生进行交流。医生能就最适合您的治疗细节提供指导。如有需要，医生还可以就酒精及物质成瘾咨询人员、互诚会或脱瘾中心，为您提供参考意见。

## ALCOHOLISM IS AN UGLY ILLNESS
## 酗酒是一种病，令人厌恶

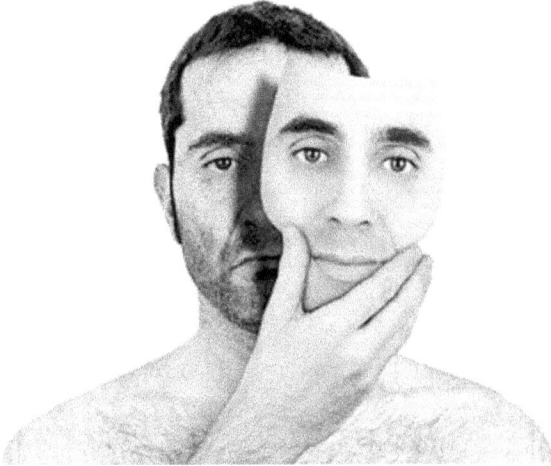

For those who know, there is no romanticizing alcoholism. It is not your drunk uncle on the holidays, and it is not the benign din of the bar room. It is the puking soiled excrement stained stupor of a man or woman who was drunk off his ass and unable to control the drinking. Drinking that may be destroying his and his family's life. It is the drunken pregnant woman maiming an unborn child. It is the mentally disabled child born to this woman months later. Lastly, it is the body in the emergency room shredded by an alcoholic who chose to drink and drive. All of these are the ugly faces of alcoholism that make us queasy and uncomfortable. These are the faces, however, staring back at us should we dare to look at the truth behind this problem. There has been a trend to window dress this horrible disease by bringing to notice the executive who is an alcoholic or the salesman who drinks too much on the weekend. Although these situations are worrisome, they come nowhere close to depicting the real ugliness of this disease. They do not show the tear stained face of the children and the wife drained of hope and stricken with misery after the death of the breadwinner who could not control his drinking. They do not do justice at all to them. Alcohol destroys lives, shatters families, and cripples generations.

对深受其害的人而言，酗酒与浪漫无关。它不是你的伯父在假日中的畅饮，也不是酒吧里令人愉悦的喧嚣。它是狂饮无度，直至不省人事的男人或女人令人作呕的呕吐污渍。酗酒可能让一个人及其家庭生活毁于一旦。是酗酒的孕妇，让未出生的孩子致残；也是她们，让数月后出生的孩子患有先天精神疾病。最终，酒驾的酗酒者，成为了急诊室里残缺不全的躯体。所有这一切，都是酗酒者的丑陋面目，令人作呕，难以接受。然而，正是这些面孔，让我们开始审视自我，看自己是否有胆量正视其背后的真相。对酗酒者或常在周末大量饮酒的销售员进行提醒，以此让更多人的人意识到这种疾病的存在，这已成为了一种趋势。尽管这些状况令人不安，但都无不与这种病态惨不忍睹的真实情况相去甚远。它们没有展现出酗酒者孩子泪痕点点的面庞和妻子的绝望，以及家庭支柱因酗酒死去时，这些家庭成员所遭遇的惨景。对于所有这些人而言，这是不公平的。酗酒毁掉了生活，令家庭支离破碎，让孩子肢体残缺。

It is a disease on par with the plague and deserves our attention in every possible way.

它是一种疾病，其危害不亚于瘟疫。值得我们以任何可能的方式，加以注意。

# You can Do It 您可以做到

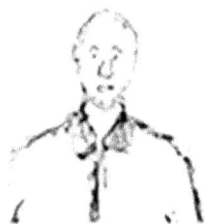

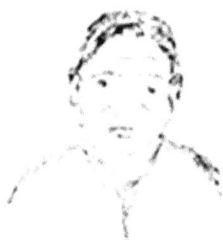

酒精中毒的特征：

肝病、肝硬化

可见及隐形的伤害

心肌症

痴呆

罹患癌症的更大风险

## YOU MIGHT BE AN ALCOHOLIC IF
### 您可能是酗酒者的前提条件

- You drink more than 4 drinks per day for women and 5 drinks per day for men.
  每日饮酒 4 次的女性，以及每日饮酒 5 次的男性；

- If you drink too many drinks in a period of 2 hours and get sick.
  如果您两小时内饮酒过量，并出现身体不适；

- If you are a man and drink more than 15 drinks per week
  如果您是每周饮酒 15 次以上的男性；

- If you are a woman and drink more than 8 drinks per week
  如果您是每周饮酒 8 次以上的女性；

- If you have blackouts. These are windows of time during drinking that you cannot remember.
  如果您出现黑朦。它通常在酗酒者无法记忆的饮酒间歇出现；

- If you drink every day
  如果您每日饮酒；

- If you start drinking in the late afternoon
  如果您总是在傍晚开始饮酒；

- If you get the shakes in the morning and need to drink to stabilize your nerves- an eye opener
  如果您在早晨出现身体颤抖，需要饮酒才能缓解神经

紧张 — 出现异常；

- If you have tried to cut down on your own because of some problems you realized
  如果您试图靠自己减少饮酒量的原因，是因为意识到了某些问题的存在；

- If you have had a fall or another accident because of drinking
  如果您因饮酒而摔倒或发生其他意外；

- If you have gotten into a fight after drinking
  如果您酒后斗殴；

- If you have committed any crime because you were drunk
  如果您因醉酒而犯罪；

- If you have medical problems due to alcoholism.
  如果您因酗酒而患病；

- If you have had a DUI ticket
  如果您因酒驾被法庭传讯。

*"We can't solve problems by using the same kind of thinking we used when we created them."* – Albert Einstein
*"用提出问题时所用到的同样思想，我们是不能解决问题的。"*
*— 阿尔伯特·爱因斯坦*

# FIRST DECISION- TO QUIT OR TO CONTROL ALCOHOL USE

## 第一个决定—戒酒或控制饮酒量

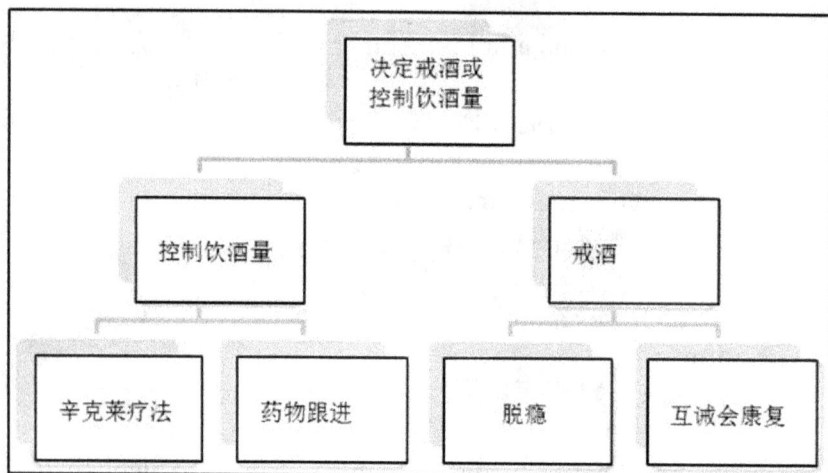

```
                    ┌─────────────┐
                    │  决定戒酒或  │
                    │  控制饮酒量  │
                    └─────────────┘
              ┌───────────┴───────────┐
        ┌──────────┐            ┌──────────┐
        │ 控制饮酒量 │            │   戒酒   │
        └──────────┘            └──────────┘
       ┌─────┴─────┐          ┌─────┴─────┐
  ┌────────┐ ┌────────┐  ┌────────┐ ┌──────────┐
  │ 辛克莱疗法│ │ 药物跟进 │  │  脱瘾  │ │ 互诚会康复 │
  └────────┘ └────────┘  └────────┘ └──────────┘
```

It seems that about 15 percent of the population is at risk of development of severe alcohol-related problems when they are exposed to it. That is a very significant number of people at risk from this very damaging illness. How do we identify those at risk and when identified, should they avoid alcohol altogether or can the alcohol use be moderated?

大约有 15%的人在接触酒精时，存在产生严重酒精相关问题的风险。这是个非常庞大的人群，他们正面临这种极具破坏性疾病的风险。我们要如何识别处于风险中的人们？何时识别？他们应该完全戒酒，还是可以适度饮酒呢？

Conventional wisdom dictates total abstinence from alcohol is the only way. Some exciting new research, however, indicates that with the help of long acting opiate blockers such as naltrexone, some may be able to moderate their use of alcohol.

一般认为彻底戒酒是唯一的办法。不过，一些新的研究令人兴奋，它们表明：借助纳曲酮之类的长效麻醉阻断剂的帮助，部分酗酒者或许能够适度饮酒。

You may be curious about what opiate receptors are. These are receptors in the brain that bind to natural opiates secreted by the brain to bring about useful effects such as controlling of pain.

您可能会好奇于什么是麻醉剂受体。大脑中的这些受体，等同于神经麻醉剂，是大脑为了产生诸如镇痛等有用效果而分泌的。

Most people, however, think that they are not in that 15 percent of the problem drinkers even when DUI tickets and the prospect of jail time is staring at them in the face. It is always the other guy that has the problem, right?

但是，绝大多数人认为自己不属于 15%的问题饮酒者中的一员，即便自己因酒驾被法庭传唤，且可能面临监禁。永远是别人在酗酒，对吗？

Be careful, lest you are one of those deniers.

不要掉以轻心，以免成为否认酗酒者中的一员。

A good clue that you may be at risk is If there is a legacy in the family of alcoholism in other family members.

如果家庭中的其他成员出现了酗酒，您可能处于这种风险之中了。这是一条有效的提示。

So first, decide if things could be better if you did not have problems related to alcohol. If you have the courage to admit that there is a problem, good for you.

因此首先，如果您还没有酗酒，要确定情况是否可以更好。如果有勇气承认自己酗酒，这对您来说是件好事。

Now you can decrease and moderate it, or you can decide to become 100 percent sober. Either way, you will need some medical support. In the next few pages, we will look at both the methods of overcoming alcohol.

现在，您可以减少饮酒量或适度饮酒，也可以决定完全戒酒。任何一种方法，都需要药物的支持。在紧接其后的内容里，我们会对摆脱酗酒的少饮酒或适度饮酒及戒酒的方法进行了解。

# You can Do It 您可以做到

## THE SINCLAIR METHOD FOR CONTROL
## 辛克莱尔控制法

This method is illustrated below.

本方法图示如下。

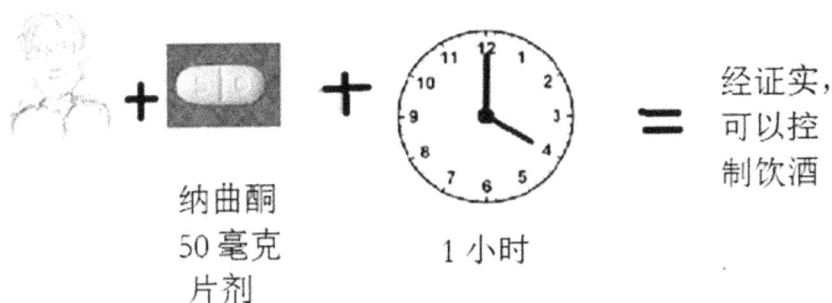

纳曲酮
50 毫克
片剂

1 小时

经证实，
可以控
制饮酒

## 减少饮酒量的辛克莱尔法

In this method, you take a Naltrexone 50 mgs tablet prescribed by a doctor one hour before taking a drink. This should be done every time you plan to have a drink for the method to succeed.

使用这种方法，你要在饮酒前一小时，服用医生

开具的处方药纳曲酮 50 毫克片剂。应该在每次打

算饮酒前，服用此药，使本方法有效。

HOW DOES IT WORK: The theory goes like this: In those with a predilection for alcohol use disorder, i.e., alcoholism, the alcohol "messes" with the opiate receptors to produce a unique, addictive response. **By blocking the opiate receptors with Naltrexone, the addiction trigger is avoided, and the person can moderate the use of alcohol and even put the drink away.**

作用机理：原理为：在经常发生酒精使用紊乱的人、即酗酒者中，酒精使麻醉剂受体出现混乱，产生出一种独特的成瘾反应。**用纳曲酮阻断麻醉剂受体，避免引起上瘾。同时，用药的人可以让酒量变得适度，甚至戒酒。**

Some who have tried this method feel that the technique has cured them of the problematic alcohol drinking. There is a famous book that goes by the name;

尝试过这种方法的一些人，感觉这种技术治愈了自己的酗酒问题。一本著名的著作，就以此法命名。

The Cure for Alcoholism: The Medically Proven Way to Eliminate Alcohol AddictionPaperback – by Roy Eskapa.

治愈酗酒：获得医疗证实的酒精脱瘾方法平装本--作者：诺依·伊斯卡帕

https://www.amazon.com/Cure-Alcoholism- Medically-Eliminate-Addiction/dp/1937856135/ref=sr_1_1?ie=UTF8&qi d=1480023191&sr=8-

1&keywords=the+alcohol+cure

There is some evidence from laboratory mice indicating that those who have had opiate blockade drink less than those rats whose opiate receptors are not blocked. Although, humans are not laboratory animals, the same opiate chemistry is shared in the brains, and the behaviors of the animal are in line with what is observed in humans who are provided opiate receptor blockade with naltrexone. They drink less alcohol. In humans, the opiate receptor genes have been implicated to the unique vulnerability of some individuals.

一些出自实验室小白鼠的证据表明，相比麻醉剂受体未经阻断的小白鼠，麻醉剂受体已阻断的小白鼠饮酒更少。尽管人不是小白鼠，但脑部麻醉化学过程是相同的；同时，小白鼠的行为，与观察使用纳曲酮阻滞麻醉剂受体的人所看到的行为是一致的。二者都减少了饮酒量。人类的麻醉剂受体基因，影响了部分个体的特有易损性。

The Sinclair method is a valid method that may benefit you. If you decide to use this method, your doctor should provide periodic checks along with any labs that may be indicated. Naltrexone has generally proven to be safe at this dosage, but occasional rises in liver enzymes are noted.

辛克莱尔法是一种行之有效的方法，可以让您获益。如果决定使用这种方法，医生应定期对您进行身体检查，并安排化验任何可能具有提示作用的指征。经证实，一般情况下，使用该剂量的纳曲酮是安全的，但偶尔也发现有肝酶升高的情况。

## TOTAL ABSTINENCE IS ACHIEVABLE AND IS THE BEST ROUTE FOR MANY

彻底戒酒是可以实现的，它也是适用于许多人的
最佳方法

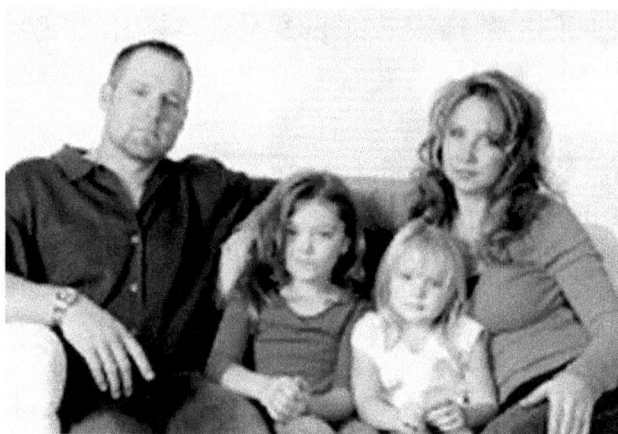

There are many individuals who are not able to moderate their drinking by any method. Their lives and their family's lives go much better when they are totally abstinent. These individuals should focus on the goal of being 100% sober and free of alcohol. It is a worthy and doable goal to be a teetotaler. Many teetotalers have found fame and success after quitting. This book discusses many ways to quit alcohol and join their ranks.

无论用任何方法，有些人都无法让自己饮酒适量。彻底戒酒后，他们及自己家庭的生活变得非常美好。这些人应该集中精力，把 100%的适度饮酒及不饮酒作为自己的目标。成为禁酒主义者，这是一个有意义、值得实现的目标。其中的许多人，已经在戒酒后实现了功成名就。本书对戒酒并跻身成功人士的多种方法进行了探讨。

You can Do It 您可以做到

# KEYS TO THE KINGDOM
## 摆脱酗酒的关键

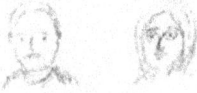

做出戒酒的决定
第 1 步

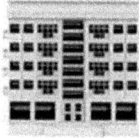

在医院或
家中脱瘾
第 2 步

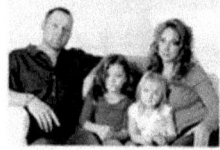

采用健康的生活方
式，适度饮酒
第 3 步

## THREE STEPS TO FREEDOM
### 摆脱酗酒三步骤

The key components are
关键要素包括：

1. Making a decision to quit
   做出戒酒的决定；

2. Getting detoxed in a safe manner at home or at a hospital or clinic under some medical supervision
   遵医嘱，以安全的方式在家或医院或脱瘾诊所脱瘾；

3. Going to AA or Secular Group meetings focused on staying sober and adopting a healthy lifestyle consistent with your values

**You can Do It 您可以做到**

加入互诚会或长期戒酒组织，全心全意地保持适度饮酒，并采用与自己价值观一致的健康生活方式。

## AN ACRONYM FOR QUITTING- F R E E D O M

### 戒酒理念缩略词--FREEDOM

One of the key things in overcoming alcohol is to make a decision to quit drinking. The FREEDOM acronym may help anchor the salient concepts for getting free

摆脱酗酒的关键之一，就是要做出戒酒的决定。FREEDOM 这个缩略词，可以帮助您固化适用于摆脱酒瘾的最重要理念。

**F-** F is for **first deciding** to quit

　　F 代表首先做出戒酒的决定；

**R-** R is for **reaching out** for help and setting a detox date

　　R 代表**寻求**帮助，并设定脱瘾日期；

**E-** E is to **expect** and visualize benefits of sobriety.

　　E 代表**充满期望，**并让戒酒的好处具体化；

**E-** E **expel** all negative influences from your life.

　　E 代表**消除**您生活中所有负面的影响因素；

**D-** D stands for **daily habit of having a quiet  time** of  15 to 20 minutes for yourself.

　　D 代表习惯于每天冥思静坐 15-20 分钟；

**O-** O **occupying yourself** with meaningful goals, hobbies, and pursuits. Be obsessed with doing what is right for you and your family.

O 代表用有意义的目标、爱好及追求**充实自己**。让自己忙于从事对自己及家庭有益的事情。

**M- Mastering Refusal Skills**

**掌握拒绝饮酒的技巧。**

## STAGES OF DETOXIFICATION
### 脱瘾各阶段介绍

Detoxification occurs over a period of about four days.

脱瘾需要大约四天的时间。

Withdrawal symptoms may begin in a matter of a few hours in a person that is a heavy alcoholic. These withdrawal symptoms may be marked by a rise in heart rate, tremulousness and a growing sense of nausea and unease. There may be strong cravings for alcohol and associated anxiety symptoms. In the next 48 hours, flushing of the face with sweating may be noticed along with an exacerbation of the features of tremulousness and tachycardia. If this is not treated, visual and auditory hallucinations may be experienced. The patient may become delirious and have a withdrawal seizure. These have previously been called rum fits. The onset of withdrawal seizures often indicates the beginning of a withdrawal delirium tremens. This can be a lethal phase with up to a 25% death rate if not treated.

停止饮酒症状大约在酗酒者停止饮酒数小时后开始出现。可能是心跳加速、发抖，以及逐渐明显的恶心与不安；也可能是饮酒冲动，及相关的焦虑症。接下来 48 小时后，可能出现脸颊潮红、出汗，并伴有颤抖及心动过速加剧。如果不治疗，可能出现幻视及幻听。患者可能变得神志昏迷，并伴有停止饮酒适应症的突然发作。这些就是之前所称的谵妄。停止饮酒症状的出现，通常表明了停止饮酒所引起的震颤性谵妄的开始。如不经治疗，可以成为致死阶段，死亡率高达 25%。

The symptoms of withdrawal can be treated easily by the use of benzodiazepines, thiamine, multivitamins and by providing adequate nutrition and hydration in a medically supervised setting where vital signs are monitored on a regular basis. Benzodiazepines are medications such as Valium, Ativan, Restoril. On the fourth and fifth day, the withdrawal symptoms subside to a significant extent. The benzodiazepines are used liberally at first to control the withdrawal symptoms. Once a stabilization dose has been reached, this is tapered down by 20 to 25% per day over the next 4 to 5 days.

停止饮酒症状可以在医院对生命体征进行常规监测的前提下，通过使用苯二氮平类药物、硫胺素、复合维生素，以及为病人补充充足的营养和含水量而轻松得到治疗。苯二氮平类药物包括安定、安定文及羟基安定。在第四和第五天，停止饮酒症状得到极大程度地减弱。初期，可以放心使用苯二氮平类药物，控制停止饮酒症状。一旦达到稳定剂量，在接下来的 4 至 5 天，每日减少用药量 20%-25%。

The thiamine prevents damage to the hippocampus and the mammillary bodies on the undersurface of the brain where memories are encoded. This damage can occur in acute alcohol withdrawal if no thiamine is provided. Before any calories in the way of dextrose solution or a meal are provided during withdrawal, it is important that thiamine is provided to the individual undergoing alcohol detox to prevent this brain damage. If it is in an emergency room,intramuscular thiamine 100 mgs is preferred. If this is not available, oral dose of 200 mgs of thiamine should suffice.

硫胺素防止对人体大脑下表面、实现记忆编码的海马体和乳头体造成损害。如果不给药硫胺素，这种损害会在突然停止饮酒时发生。如果在停止饮酒期间，采用了脱瘾疗法，那么，在补充热量或进食前，给药硫胺素，对于个体脱瘾，防止大脑损伤至关重要。如果在急诊室，最好采用肌注硫胺素 100 毫克。如果无法实施肌注，口服 200 毫克也可满足疗效。

## LET'S TAKE A LOOK NOW AT SOME OF THE 50 WAYS OF OVERCOMING ALCOHOL

让我们立刻了解一下摆脱酗酒的各种方法吧！

# You can Do It 您可以做到

## WAY 1
## 方法 1

### THE DAWNING OF INSIGHT: ALL OF A SUDDEN AND AT ONCE- A TRUE EUREKA MOMENT!!
出现深刻认知：出乎意料、突然出现—一个真正的尤里卡时刻

Sometimes, the individual can have a truly moving experience of sudden insight that shakes the soul and allows one to see for a flash moment the totality of one's life situation. This vision allows one to see alcohol and its wickedness for what it is and also shows a path out. The founder of Alcoholic Anonymous [AA] Bill Wilson had such an insight. He, later on, shared his experience with others. His sincerity and abiding dedication to the welfare of others that were suffering from alcohol helped build the AA community into the single greatest force for overcoming alcoholism.

有时，个体的深层认知会猛然出现真实地变化，意识发生动摇，让人瞬间看到自己的整体生活状况。这种认识，让人可以看清酗酒及其危害性，让抽身而出的光明之路得以显现。匿名酗酒者组织[互诚会]的创始人比尔·维尔森，就有过这样的深刻认识。随后，他与其他人分享了自己的经历。真诚与为承受酗酒之痛的其他人谋求幸福的不懈奉献，帮助他把这个互诚会，建设成为了一个最具影响力的摆脱酗酒社区。

Many others have had this insight and you can too. This insight can lead to a profound revulsion for alcohol.

许多人已经具有了这样的深刻认识，您也可以。这种认识可以让您对酗酒产生强烈反感，意义深远。

# WAY 2
## 方法 2

### ACHIEVING INSIGHT: THE BUMPY AND GRADUAL PROCESS
让认知变为现实：循序渐进的曲折过程

For others, the accumulation of insight and wisdom is the gift of past failures. This insight gradually grows and reaches a tipping point at which a decision is made by the alcoholic to quit.

对于其他人而言，深刻认识与智慧的累积，是曾经的挫折所给予的馈赠。这种认识逐渐发展，达到成熟。这时，个体做出停止饮酒的决定。

If you have experienced pain from alcohol, you can take this pain and make a decision to take concrete steps towards ridding yourself off this malady. This can include steps such as setting a date, removing all alcoholic drinks from home and scheduling an appointment with the doctor. The doctor may then admit you to a detox center or can make arrangements for detox at home or another facility.

如果经历过酗酒带来的痛苦，您可以接受这种痛苦，并做出决定，采取切实的步骤，摆脱这种病态。可以包含的步骤如：设定停止饮酒日期、丢掉家中的所有酒精饮料，以及安排时间咨询医生。那时，医生或许会让您进入脱瘾中心接受帮助，或者在家里或其他机构进行脱瘾治疗。

You can Do It 您可以做到

# WAY 3
# 方法 3

## BY SCIENTIFICALLY WEIGHING THE BENEFITS AND RISKS, THE PROS AND CONS - AND DECIDING TO QUIT
## 科学权衡得失与利弊 — 决定戒酒

This is a deliberate exercise of looking at the benefits and risks from alcohol use. Most of the so-called benefits are not really benefits.

分析酗酒的利与弊，这是一种刻意地锻炼。绝大部分所谓的利，都不是真正的利。

| Supposed Benefit<br>可能的利 | Reality<br>现实 | Risks<br>弊 |
|---|---|---|
| **Myth:**<br>**It improves**<br>**Relationships**<br>错误认知：<br>饮酒可以拉近关系 | Reality:<br>It is often the cause of arguments and fights.<br>现实：<br>饮酒通常会造成争执与斗殴 | Risks:<br>Arguments and fights may lead to arrests, broken Relationships<br>弊：<br>争执与斗殴可能导致入狱，关系破裂 |
| **Myth: It has**<br>**health**<br>**benefits**<br>错误认知：<br>饮酒有助于健康 | Reality: It reduces life expectancy by at least a decade. Sober | Risks: There is a risk for liver disease, cirrhosis, heart disease and |

43

| | people live longer<br>现实：它至少使寿命缩短 10 年。适度饮酒的人寿命更长。 | dementia.<br>弊：存在患肝病、肝硬化、心脏病和痴呆的风险。 |
|---|---|---|

| Myth: It is useful for reducing anxiety<br>错误认知：有助于减少焦虑 | Reality: Alcohol may help in the short term but increases anxiety in the long term and also causes depression.<br>现实：酗酒可能有助于短期的焦虑减少。但就长期而言，会增加焦虑，并引起精神抑郁。 | Risks: Alcohol may cause one to have greater impairment from anxiety and depression<br>弊：酗酒可以让一个人因焦虑和抑郁，受到更大的伤害。 |
|---|---|---|
| Myth: It can be used safely at work or in travel<br>错误认知：工作或出行时饮酒是安全的。 | Reality: Alcohol is the number one cause of serious accidents on the road, water, and in the air<br>现实：酗酒是严重道路交通事故、水上交通事故及空中交通事故的首因。 | Risks: You along with someone else may be killed in an accident caused by alcohol<br>弊：其他人可能和您一起死于酗酒造成的意外事故。 |
| Myth: It can be used safely in low amounts during pregnancy<br>错误认知：孕期少量 | No amount of alcohol is safe during pregnancy for the child.<br>现实：对于胎儿而言 | Fetal alcohol syndrome is a well-known risk from alcohol use by the pregnant |

44

# You can Do It 您可以做到

| 饮酒是安全可靠的。 | ，母体在孕期饮酒，任何量都是不安全的。 | mother<br>弊：致命的酗酒并发症，这种总所周知的风险，是因怀孕母亲酗酒带来的。 |
|---|---|---|

# WAY 4
方法 4

## BY PROMISING A LOVED ONE TO QUIT FOR THEM AND SETTING A DETOX DATE
承诺为所爱的人戒酒，并设定脱瘾日期

Some individuals are truly shaken by the amount of emotional trauma that they've caused their family and children or their loved one. They make them a promise to quit and honor that promise and that love by setting up a stop date. They then consult with a doctor and arrange to get detoxed. This is usually by admission to a hospital for 4 to 5 days. If they are going to do an outpatient detox with help from the doctor, they will go on to get food, water and any medications ordered plus any vitamins needed such as thiamine for use during detoxification. Their doctor, nurse practitioner or other medical provider experienced with outpatient detox will provide them further instructions.

事实上，有些人会因自己酗酒而为家庭、子女或 爱人造成的巨大情感创伤，深感内疚。他们向家人承诺戒酒，并设定戒酒日期，以此表达对这份承诺和亲情的尊重。之后，他们会咨询医生并做出安排，完成脱瘾治疗。通常，医生会让他们住院 4 至 5 天。如果打算在医生的帮助下，进行门诊脱瘾，就继续进食、饮水，并按要求服药，以及服用脱瘾治疗期间所需服用的维生素，如硫胺素。具有门诊脱瘾经验的医生、护理人员或其他医疗服务人员，会为这些人提供进一步的指导。

## WAY 5
## 方法 5

# BY GRADUALLY REDUCING ALCOHOL INTAKE DUE TO AN ULTIMATUM FROM THE BOSS
## 上司的最后通牒，迫使酗酒者逐渐减少饮酒量

Some individuals have successfully weaned themselves off alcohol when they felt their job was jeopardized. This is often triggered by an ultimatum from the boss. The boss should also have referred the individual for help through EAP (Employee Assistance Program). If he did not, know that this exists at most places of employment. You can ask the personnel department about the contact information for EAP. They usually have a toll free line and are trained to be very sympathetic, polite and helpful. Anything you share with EAP is confidential and not shared with your employer. If you are wise, you will avail of help that is available through EAP before the ultimatum and threat to your employment arrives.

有些人感觉到自己的工作因饮酒而受到危害时，戒酒成功。通常，上司的最后通牒促使其戒酒。上司还应通过 EAP（员工帮助计划），为员工提供帮助。尚未实施 EAP 计划的老板，应知道绝大部分企业都履行该计划。您可以向单位人事部门索要 EAP 的联系方式。通常，他们都有单位人员名单，服务热情周到、待人礼貌，乐于助人。您提供给 EAP 的任何信息，他们都会保密，而不与雇主分享。如果是个聪明人，您会在老板的最后通牒和威胁到来前，利用好 EAP 提供的帮助。

## WAY 6
## 方法 6

## BY FINDING OBJECTIVE EVIDENCE IN LABORATORY RESULTS OF THE DAMAGE BEING CAUSED TO YOUR BODY

从化验结果中找出酗酒有害于身体的客观证据

When you visit your doctor the next time, ask about the laboratory results. If there are swollen red blood cells as indicated by increased MCV (mean corpuscular volume) or elevated liver enzymes, it should start ringing an alarm bell for you. There may be other associated abnormalities such as a low B12 level due to malabsorption. You can ask the doctor for help in overcoming your alcohol problems when you are told about these findings.

再次就诊时，您可以向医生了解，提示酗酒对身体造成损害的化验室结果包含哪些。如果有 MCV（红细胞平均容量）增加或肝酶升高提示的红细胞肿大，那就是对您的警告。可能存在其他的关联异常，比如因吸收不良而造成的维生素 B12 降低。获知这些化验结果后，您可以就摆脱酗酒向医生寻求帮助。

# You can Do It 您可以做到

## WAY 7
## 方法 7

## MODERATION BY NOT DRINKING TWO DAYS IN A ROW
不连续饮酒，使饮酒量适度

You can reduce the damage caused by alcohol by not drinking every day. If you can skip a day, it will be less toxic to your liver and other body organs. It means, if you drink on Monday, then skip Tuesday before drinking on Wednesdays.

您可以不要每天饮酒，以此降低酒精对身体造成的伤害。如果少喝一天，酒精对您肝脏和其他器官的毒害就少一些。这意味着如果您周一饮酒，那么周二就不喝，周三再喝。

On the day you are going to drink, take a Naltrexone 50 mg tablet an hour before you plan to drink.

在打算饮酒的当天，提前一小时服用纳曲酮 50 毫克片剂。

Other ways to moderate drinking is to sip slowly and eat food when you drink. Also, limit yourself to 2 to 3 drinks at the most.

让酒量适度的其他方法包括少量慢饮，同时进食。此外，将自己的饮酒次数限制在最多 2 至 3 次。

This strategy will reduce the total amount of alcohol used and avoid dangerous rises in alcohol levels.

这种办法使总的饮酒量减少，避免因过量而发生危险。

# WAY 8
## 方法 8

## BY RECOGNIZING THAT DRINKING IS LIKE LICKING HONEY OFF A RAZOR BLADE FOR SOME
### 认识到酗酒无异于铤而走险

酗酒犹如铤而走险。

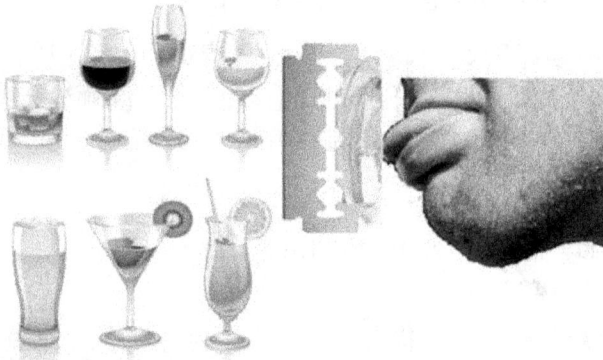

DRINKING ALCOHOL IS LIKE TRYING TO LICK HONEY FROM A RAZOR BLADE

If you are someone at high risk due to a strong family history of alcoholism or past problems with alcohol, you by definition cannot safely drink alcohol. You should aim for total abstinence. You can consider moderated use with the help of naltrexone. Unprotected exposure to alcohol would be like trying to lick honey from a razor blade. You will get hurt.

如果因明显的家族酗酒史，或曾出现酗酒问题，您有酗酒的高风险。那对您而言，饮酒绝对是不安全的。因此，您的目标应该是彻底戒酒。在服用纳曲酮的情况下，您可以考虑适度饮酒。饮酒而不采取任何保护措施，无异于铤而走险。您将因此受到伤害。

## WAY 9
## 方法 9

### BY DECIDING TO REMOVE ALCOHOLIC DRINKS FROM THE HOME, OFFICE AND VEHICLE

决定扔掉家中、办公室和车内的酒精饮料

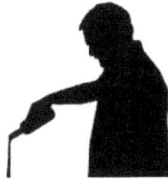

When you realize that you have had enough of the alcohol and related problems, the wisest thing you can do is to get detoxed and at the same time, get rid of the remaining alcohol from your home, work, and vehicle. Any stashes in the garage or the barn should also be removed. Knowing that no alcohol is available can reduce the urges and cravings for using it. By making the home environment safe and free of alcohol, your chance of maintaining sobriety is greatly improved. Get rid of all of it.

当意识到自己大量饮酒，并出现相关问题时，您最明智的作法是摆脱酒瘾。同时，扔掉家里、办公场所和车内剩余的酒。存放在车库或储藏室的所有酒，也都该扔掉。懂得不喝酒，生活照旧，这可以降低饮酒的冲动与强烈愿望。让家成为没有酒的安全环境，您保持滴酒不沾的机会就大大增加了。扔掉所有的酒，一滴不剩。

## WAY 10

方法 10

## BY TELLING A FEW TRUSTED FRIENDS AND FAMILY MEMBERS ABOUT YOUR PLAN TO DETOX AND QUIT

把脱瘾及戒酒计划告诉值得信赖的朋友及家人

This strategy can help you stay committed to your goal. Your friends and family members can also take extra steps not to bring in alcohol into the home or to offer it to you if they are sincere in their friendship or kinship. No friend or family member will ever compromise the goals of someone in this situation who is trying to overcome alcohol.

这种方法可以让您信守承诺，实现目标。朋友和家人还可以采取其他的步骤，比如不把酒带回家，或者不向你提供酒。前提是他们忠于自己的友情或亲情。身为朋友或家人的任何人，都不会在您努力摆脱酗酒、实现目标时拖后腿。

# WAY 11
## 方法 11

## BY FIGURING OUT WHAT LED TO THE LAST RELAPSE
找出导致最终故态复萌的原因所在

After detox, it will be all important to maintain your sobriety and to prevent a relapse. It is wise to have examined and recognized the triggers that had led to your relapse in the past. With this knowledge, you can plan to remove those relapse triggers from your environment. You should also make plans on how to deal with them should they come up again.

脱瘾后，保持不饮酒，防止重新上瘾，这非常重要。审视并认识到之前导致自己故态复萌的诱因，这是明智之举。有了这种认知，您就可以计划去除身边的那些令您故态复萌的诱因了。此外，您还应制定计划，应对诱因再次出现。

# WAY 12
## 方法 12

## BY COMMITTING TO A BIGGER GOAL IN YOUR LIFE
承诺实现更高远的人生目标

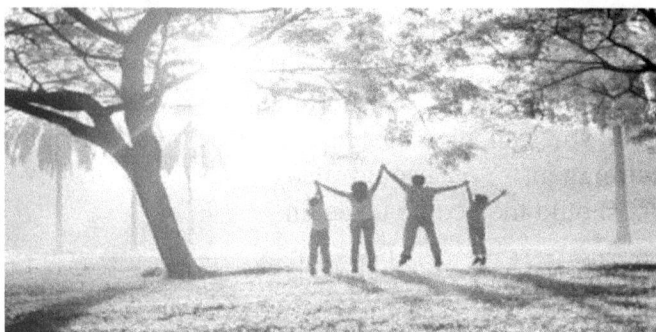

It is important sometimes to set bigger goals for your life. Some individuals are frustrated about not having realized their life's goals. They have always been told to be practical and to settle for less in their lives. If they are talented, this can be a blow to their sense of well-being. If you fall into this category, you can benefit from individual therapy or a life coach who provides you a plan to achieve bigger goals in your life. The setting of such bigger goals can help lift you out of your depression, help you make a decision to get detoxed and get sober.

有时，为自己的人生设定更远大的目标，这事关重大。生活没有目标，这让有些人萎靡不振。总有人告诉他们立足现实，对生活的目标低一些。如果天资聪慧，他们的幸福感会因此而受挫。如果您就是其中一员，可以从个体疗法中获得帮助，或者受益于人生导师的帮助。人生导师帮助您指定计划，实现人生更远大的目标。设定更远大的目标，可以帮助您摆脱抑郁情绪，

# You can Do It 您可以做到

有助于您做出决定，远离酗酒，适度饮酒。

## WAY 13
## 方法 13

## BY SEPARATING FROM TOXIC RELATIONSHIPS
远离酒友

If you are involved in a toxic relationship, it can sap your strength, motivation and in general, make your life a living hell filled with anxiety and depression. Such depression and anxiety states are the breeding grounds for alcohol, self-defeating behaviors of alcoholism and other addictions.

如果卷入到一种有害的交往中，您的优势会削弱，积极性会降低。总体而言，它会让您的生活一团糟，充满焦虑与抑郁情绪。这种抑郁与焦虑状态，会滋生酗酒，以及因酗酒及其他上瘾所导致的自我挫败行为。

The key to your recovery may, therefore, be to let go of a relationship that is not working despite your best efforts.

因此，摆脱其影响的关键，可能是结束这种关系。因为即便付出最大努力，也无法让这种关系对您有利。

It is better to let go of relationships than to throw your life away in self-defeating behaviors. When the wounds of the relationship heal, your mood will lift, and you will have a greater chance of recovery from alcohol-related problems.

与对自我挫败行为放任自流相比，结束这种关系更好。当这种关系所造成的伤痛痊愈时，您的心情会变好，摆脱酗酒的机会更大。

You can Do It 您可以做到

# WAY 14
## 方法 14

## BY PRACTICING AND USING REFUSAL SKILLS
练习并运用拒绝劝酒的技巧

You will be tempted to take "one last drink" or to take a drink "for old times' sake" or some other dumb rationalization.

"最后一杯"、"为老交情"喝一杯，或其他一些愚蠢的理由，都会成为您喝酒的诱惑。

## DO NOT FALL FOR THESE PLOYS
不要陷入这些计谋之中

Practice saying out aloud in a firm but in a cordial manner, "I am sorry, I cannot accept the drink due to doctor's recommendation."

练习以诚恳的方式，郑重地大声说出："抱歉，是医生建议我不饮酒。"

There are many conditions that are made worse by alcohol such as heart disease, liver disease, and mood disorders. There is also an increased risk of certain cancers. You can truthfully say that your doctor has advised you not to use alcohol for health reasons. You don't have to go into details. There are some medications also such as metronidazole or Antabuse, and others that cannot be combined with alcohol.

因为饮酒而让身体每况愈下的情形很多。比如心脏出现问题，患肝病，以及情绪失控。还会增加特定癌症的患病风险。您可

## You can Do It 您可以做到

以无比真诚地表示，出于健康原因，医生已建议您不要饮酒，而不必赘述细节。此外，有些药物，如甲硝哒唑或安塔布斯，以及其他药物也不能在饮酒期间服用。

You can offer such valid excuses truthfully and get yourself out of the situation. You should feel comfortable saying this because would not be lying. Be sure to practice this in front of the mirror.

您可以诚实地说出类似的正当理由，让自己脱身。做出这样的表达，您应该感到安心。因为这不是撒谎。一定要面对镜子练习。

By practicing and using refusal skills when someone offers you a drink, you increase the chances of staying sober.

练习和运用拒绝饮酒的技巧，您就能在有人劝酒时，增加自己适度饮酒的机会。

You can also tell them that you are committed to your sobriety and to not offer you drinks in the future.

此外，您还可以告诉他们，自己要戒酒，请他们以后不要再劝你喝酒了。

There is no need to be apologetic about making such statements.

做出这样的表述，您无需感到歉意。

You should avoid the company of those that try to push alcohol on you despite your efforts.

对已说明缘由，仍试图劝酒的人，应避免交往。

# Overcoming Alcohol 摆脱酗酒

# You can Do It 您可以做到

## WAY 15
## 方法 15

## BY HAVING A BUDDY WITH YOU IN A RISKY SITUATION
## 让好友陪你出席有过量饮酒风险的场合

It's good to have a friend that is committed to your staying sober accompany you if you're going to be in a situation where there is a risk for relapse. This person can back you up when needed and steer you away if needed.

当去的地方，存在让您重新酗酒的风险，那么，让一位可以让您保持饮酒适度的朋友相伴，这是个不错的决定。这个人可以在需要时，为您提供支持，并在需要时带您抽身离开。

## WAY 16
## 方法 16

### BY RECOGNIZING THAT THE GLAMOR OF DRINKING IS FALSE ADVERTISING

认识到对饮酒美妙感受的描绘，都是华而不实的广告用语

You should recognize that most of the debonair actors or actresses that you see on TV and the silver screen are paid to act in a certain way. They act to portray popular misconceptions about alcohol as being sexy, classy or attractive. The fact is that drinking does not make anyone more attractive or glamorous. Drinking, in fact, dulls the senses and makes the individual seemed dependent and needy.

Some of these actors who tried to take their acting into real life ended up with terrible alcohol-related problems. For some, it cost them their life. Hence recognize that alcohol advertisements are designed to sell liquor. In real life, alcohol will add no glamor to your life but may bring many problems.

您应认识到电视和电影中看到的、酒后温文尔雅的男主角或女主角，都是得到报酬，以特定方式而作的表演。他们的表演，表现了与饮酒有关、大行其道的错误理念，即饮酒使人性感、优雅或富有魅力。事实是，饮酒不会让任何人变得更具吸引力，或富有魅力。实际上，它会让人感觉迟钝，可能产生酒精依赖，而且生活陷入困境。试图让自己的表演与真实的生活融为一体的那些演员中，有些人最终出现了可怕的酗酒问题。其中一些，甚至为此失去了生命。因此，要认识到酒广告，都是为了销售酒而设计的。在现实生活中，酒不仅不能为您增添魅力，还会带来诸多问题。

## WAY 17
## 方法 17

# BY REALIZING THAT DRINKING OF EXCESSIVE ALCOHOL DOES NOT MAKE A MAN MORE MANLY
## 意识到过量饮酒不会让男人更有魅力

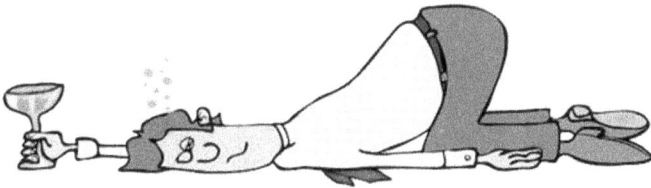

There is a popular misconception that a man is stronger in some way if he can drink a large amount of alcohol. The fact is that it does not matter if you are a puny hundred pound weakling or if you are a WWF pro wrestler. Your vital internal organs are not protected by the muscle mass on the outside. The heavy drinker causes a greater degree of liver damage, heart toxicity, and brain damage. The insane notion of proving manliness by drinking to excess is particularly dangerous if the individual is vain and insecure. He may try to impress others by drinking heavily. In a cruel twist of irony, such heavy drinking may have a toxic effect on the male sex organs and lead to impotence.

认为如果男人酒量大，就从某种程度上代表其身体更加强壮，这是一种常见的误解。事实上，酒量大小与您是否区区百磅、身形弱小，或是否是职业摔跤手毫无关系。人体重要的内部器官，不是由身体外部大块的肌肉保护的。酗酒，会引起更剧烈的肝脏损伤、心脏中毒及脑部受损。如果一个人自高自大且缺乏自信，通过过量饮酒，证明自己具有男人魅力的疯狂想法就尤其危险。因为他可能借助过度饮酒，让他人对自己印象深刻。

极具讽刺意味的是，这种过度饮酒可能对男性性器官造成毒副作用，导致阳痿。

# WAY 18
## 方法 18

## BY REJECTING THE MYTH THAT BEING AN ALCOHOLIC IS A SIGN OF ARTISTIC TALENT
### 对酗酒象征艺术天赋这一谬论嗤之以鼻

Some writers, actors, and poets have been known to have problems with alcohol. Just like anyone else, they may have emotional issues that they try to resolve through their art. They may also try to use alcohol in part to self-medicate their issues. The alcohol molecule, however, does not know that they are a writer, actor or poet and traps them into the trap that is alcoholism just like it entraps others. The artist may believe the myth about alcohol and art and may use this as an excuse to justify their own use whether it is relevant to their situation or not. They just got trapped into alcoholism and are looking for any justification to continue like any other person in denial. This is justification by the alcoholic in them and not the need of the artist or writer. Hubris and false pride is a dangerous thing and a bigger trap in many ways. This psychological trap along with the physiological trap of alcoholism can be a real challenge. The distorted thinking caused by pride makes them blind to the reality that anyone who combines depression, anxiety, and alcohol is likely to become an alcoholic. They are not an alcoholic because they are an artist. If you are an alcoholic or artist and have alcohol-related problems, realize that the risk for alcoholism is the same for you as it is for others. You can also overcome the problems just like others can. You will be a greater artist, a better writer if you attain sobriety or moderated drinking that is not toxic to you.

众所周知，一些作家、演员和诗人酗酒。同其他人一样，他们可能碰到了情感问题，并试图通过艺术加以解决。此外，他们可能在一定程度上，试图借助酗酒反思自己的问题。但酒分子并不知道他们是作家、演员或诗人，同样让他们深陷其中难以自拔，就如同让其他人上瘾一样。艺术家可能对酗酒与艺术间的这种谬误深信不疑，也可能把它当作一种借口，证明无论境况如何，酗酒都是正当的。他们不过是陷于其中无力自拔，并为这种行为寻求正当理由，以便继续像不承认酗酒有害的其他人一样执迷不悟。这是他们酗酒的正当理由，而不是作为艺术家或作家的需求。狂妄自大与虚荣是危险的。某种程度而言，这是更大的陷阱。这种心理陷阱，同酗酒的心理陷阱一起，可以成为真正的挑战。同时出现情绪抑郁、焦虑，并热衷饮酒的任何人，具有酗酒的可能性。而妄自尊大所带来的错误认识，会使人对这一事实视而不见。他们会认为自己是艺术家，所以不是酒鬼。如果您酗酒，或是一名艺术家，并出现了与饮酒相关的问题，要意识到酗酒对于您的风险，与它对于其他人的风险是一样的。而且，正如其他人可以摆脱酒瘾一样，您也可以战胜它。如果戒酒或适度饮酒，不让自己深受其害，您就可以成为更伟大的艺术家。

You don't have to make yourself physically sick in order to create art. You should have the courage to feel deeply and express yourself without resorting to any type of crutches.

为了创作艺术，您不必让自己的身体承受病痛，而应该有勇气，深刻地感受并表达自己，不要求助于任何类型的物质支持。

If you are prominent, you can become an advocate for sobriety and even be a guiding light for other artists that may be floundering in confusion. You can model sobriety to others that are not artists but look up to you. Such altruistic acts will also help you in your life in many told and untold ways.

如果您富有影响力，可以成为戒酒倡导者，甚至成为其他可能尚在困顿迷惑中挣扎的艺术家们的指路明灯。对于不是艺术家，

## You can Do It 您可以做到

但仰慕您的其他人而言，您可以成为戒酒模范。这种无私的行为，也会让您在生活中诸多已知及未知的方面，受益匪浅。

## WAY 19
## 方法 19

# BY GIVING UP THE NEED FOR TOXIC SYMPATHY FROM OTHERS
### 放弃向他人索取毫无意义同情的需求

There are some alcoholics who will try to act funny in their drunken state. Alcoholism is a serious disease and is not funny or humorous. The antics of the drunk are to be pitied rather than taken as comedy. Some alcoholics will seek to gain sympathy from their sodden misery. Although it is ok to give them a shoulder to cry on, the alcoholic can become dependent on the sympathies garnered by their sick role. Such sympathies alone are never enough to cure the person. It can mislead and encourage the person to continue their drinking in order to continue getting sympathy or disapproval from others. Some have a need to see themselves be put down in a twist of masochism. If you are negating yourself in order to receive such sympathy, know that it is not helpful to you and that you have a better life awaiting you. Such tokens of passing sympathy are like the dimes and cents given to a panhandler that allows him to buy his next few beer. Let go of such toxic sympathy and attain your sobriety.

一些酗酒者，会试图让自己在醉酒时的表现有趣。

但酗酒是一种严重的病，不具有趣味或幽默感。醉酒者的怪异举止，值得同情，但不会被看作是滑稽表演。另一些酗酒者，则会寻求获得他人对自己污渍满身的惨状的同情。尽管为他们提供宣泄时的依靠，这是正确的，但他们会对以病态而博得同情具有依赖性。要治愈一个人的伤痛，仅有这种同情，是永远不够的。它会让人误入歧途，并对继续博得他人同情或排斥形成鼓励。一些人需要看到他人制止自己自虐。如果您为了得到这样的同情而否定自己，要知道那无对您没有帮助。而且，更美好的生活正在等待着您。这种传递同情的作法，无异于对乞丐的施舍，让他可以再一次买到少得可怜的啤酒。让这种有弊无利的同情滚蛋，实现戒酒。

# WAY 20
# 方法 20

## BY BEING INSPIRED BY THE EXAMPLE OF THOSE THAT GAVE UP ALCOHOL
受到成功戒酒典范人物的感召

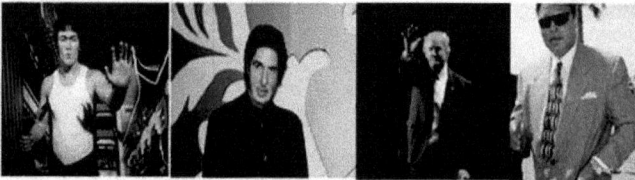

李小龙　　阿米塔布·巴沙坎　　唐纳德·特朗普　　穆罕默德·阿里

Images purchased from Dreamtime.com

© Americanspirit | Dreamstime.com · <a href="https://www.dreamstime.com/editorial-

**TEETOTALER POWERHOUSES**

A person may be inspired by some great people that have never used alcohol or have given it up and become teetotalers. This list includes luminaries such as the following:

有些知名人士从不饮酒，或已戒酒并成为了禁酒主义者，酗酒者可以受到这些人的感召。如下这张名单，就包含了其中的杰出人物：

Bruce Lee, Legendary Martial Arts,

Fighter Mahatma Gandhi, Great Freedom Fighter Donald Trump, President of USA

Amitabh Bachchan, iconic Bollywood actor.

李小龙，传奇武打明星；斗士圣人甘地；杰出的自由斗士、美

# You can Do It 您可以做到

国总统唐纳德·特朗普；阿米塔布·巴沙坎，印度宝莱坞偶像男演员

Alec Baldwin, Hollywood actor Mohammed Ali, World Boxing Champion Billy Graham, Famous Evangelist

Jennifer Lopez, Singer, Actress

亚力克·鲍德温，好莱坞男演员

默罕默德·阿里，世界拳王

比利·格拉哈姆，知名福音传道者

Larry Ellison, Billionaire CEO of Oracle Joe Biden, Vice President of USA

Don Bradman, legendary cricketer

百万富豪拉瑞·艾莉森，甲骨文公司 CEO；乔·拜登，美国副总统

唐·布莱德曼，传奇板球队员

Anil Ambani, wealthy industrialist, investor and humanitarian

安尼尔·安巴尼，富有的实业家、投资人和人道主义者

There are many more great men and women.

还有更多伟大的男性与女性。

More information about other teetotalers can be found at this link.

https://en.wikipedia.org/wiki/List_of_teetotalers

点击以下链接，可以获取与其他禁酒主义者有关的更多信息：
https://en.wikipedia.org/wiki/List_of_teetotalers

# WAY 21
## 方法 21

## BY EXAMINING YOUR LIFE IN A CATHARTIC THERAPY SETTING

用宣泄疗法审视自己

Catharsis is a process of emptying and letting go. Some individuals may benefit from psychotherapy that addresses their underlying issues and anxieties in this type of therapy. It can bring up old repressed anxieties and the process of letting go of past emotional baggage can be very liberating. Often, such anxieties take root in childhood trauma, deprivations or abuse. This therapy can be combined with journaling. This is the process of simply writing about your feelings about the past or future in a journal. This journal should be kept confidential and can even be destroyed at the end of the successful conclusion of the therapy. Sometimes it can be preserved if the individual chooses to do so.

宣泄是放空思想与摒弃杂念的过程。有些人可能从这类心理疗法中获益。该疗法解决的是人的潜在问题和焦虑。它会触及曾经得到抑制的焦虑，并让过去的情绪负担得到彻底地释放。通常，这种焦虑的根源是儿童时期所承受的伤痛、被剥夺或受虐。治疗可与记日记相结合。即治疗过程中，用日记简要记录自己对过去或未来的感受。这本日记应该得到妥善保管，它会在治疗得出成功结论后销毁。有时，如果个体选择保留日记，也可以保存下来。

# WAY 22
# 方法 22

## WITH AA AND SELF-HELP GROUPS- MEETING REGULARLY WITH OTHERS WHO WANT TO QUIT

参加互诚会及自助戒酒组织，定期与希望戒酒的

其他人聚会

Having the right company can have a very uplifting effect on your mood and motivation to do better in your life. AA meetings are based on this model of gathering likeminded people who have the one single goal- abstinence from alcohol. These groups can be a god send if you want to quit alcohol. The mutual commitment by the members to sobriety is assuring and encouraging. Individuals that are struggling can learn from the struggles of others and receive help and comfort from others. The more mature members serve as living manifestations of the truth that it is possible to achieve sobriety and stay sober. Self-help groups have helped many individuals achieve sobriety and a healthier lifestyle. They can help you too. You will benefit if you make these groups a cornerstone of your sober life style.

拥有正确的同伴，可以对您的情绪产生积极影响，

并让您更加积极地把生活变得更美好。互诚会采

用的主要模式，是让把戒酒作为唯一目标、有类似想法的人聚在一起。如果您希望戒酒，这些组织可以成为绝佳的选择。成员彼此承诺戒酒，这成为了一种相互的保证及鼓励。充当事实见证者的成员越成熟，互诚会越有可能成功地让参与者戒酒及适度饮酒。自助戒酒组织已经帮助许多人成功戒酒，拥有了更加健康的生活方式。因此，他们也可以为您提供帮助。如果让这个组织成为您适度饮酒生活方式的转折点，您会获益。

You can Do It 您可以做到

## WAY 23
## 方法 23

## WITH THE HELP OF PROFESSIONALLY LED GROUP THERAPY

借助专业引导下的群体疗法的帮助

Alcohol and drug counselors are trained to provide therapy, guidance, education, motivation, and support for those individuals that want to quit. They are also trained in group dynamics and can facilitate and move the group towards their jointly shared goals of attaining sobriety. Sometimes, they may be recovered alcoholics or drug users and have an enhanced understanding and empathy for the struggles of the alcoholic. You may find such groups in your community by a search on google or the yellow pages. Insurance plans cover such treatment. They are very helpful for consolidating your recovery.

酒精与毒品滥用咨询员都经过培训，可以为希望

戒酒的人员，提供治疗、引导、指导、激励及支

持。他们还接受过群体动态培训，可以促使并让

群体向实现戒酒的共有目标发展。有时，他们可

能身处酗酒或吸毒者中间，更深刻地理解及同情

酗酒者为此进行的抗争。登录谷歌搜索或查询电话号码簿，您可能会在所在社区，找到这样的群体。保险计划可以支付这种治疗的费用。这些群体非常有助于您巩固康复。

## WAY 24
## 方法 24

## BY GRADUAL REDUCTION AND TAPERING OF THE AMOUNT OF ALCOHOL USED DAILY

逐渐减少每日饮酒量并逐渐戒酒

Theoretically, you can taper yourself off by gradually cutting down your alcohol intake in consultation with your doctor. A family member or friend should be present with you during the detox. During the detox, the use of oral vitamins such as thiamine 100 milligrams per day and multivitamins is essential to prevent adverse neurological events. The detox can be achieved by the gradual reduction over 5 to 10 days. For a five day detox, the amount of alcohol is reduced by 1/5 every day. So if you take five drinks per day, you would start with five drinks on day 1, four on day 2, three on day 3, two on day 4 and one on day 5.

理论上来说，您可以咨询医生，通过逐渐减少饮酒量，让自己逐渐戒酒。脱瘾期间，您应该有一位家庭成员或朋友相伴。脱瘾过程中，每日口服维生素，如硫胺素 100 毫克，及复合维生素至关重要，可以防止神经学疾病的出现。5 至 10 天后，饮酒量逐渐减少，由此实现脱瘾。对于一次为期五天的脱瘾治疗，每天减少的饮酒量为原酒量的 1/5。因此，如果您每天饮酒五次，脱瘾治疗将从第一天饮酒五次开始，然后是第二天四次，第三天三次，第四天两次，直至第五天一次。

If the person experiences hallucinations, confusion or fits (seizures), 911 should be called and person moved to a hospital setting.

如果出现幻觉、神志不清或痉挛（癫痫），应拨打急救电话

911，并将病人送至医院接受治疗。

You can Do It 您可以做到

## WAY 25
## 方法 25

## BY TREATING UNDERLYING DEPRESSION WITH MEDICATIONS AND THERAPY

用药物和疗法治疗潜在抑郁症

Almost all alcoholics become depressed. This depression takes away the motivation, the drive, and energy and will to do anything. With sobriety, most alcohol induced depression goes away in about 4 to 6 weeks.

几乎所有的酗酒者都会变得抑郁。这种抑郁令其面对任何事情时，丧失积极性、没有动力，萎靡不振并看不到希望。通过戒酒，因酗酒而引起的绝大部分抑郁情绪，会在约 4 至 6 周后消失殆尽。

If you still suffer from significant depressive symptoms after a period of 4 to 6 weeks or have had previous episodes of serious depression that was treated with antidepressants, you should ask the doctor to consider antidepressant medications for you. Effective treatment of depression can have a life- changing effect. It has been described as being akin to the turning on of a light in a dark room. Sometimes if one antidepressant does not work, another may work better. A psychiatrist or a family doctor who is informed about mental health issues can prescribe the antidepressant.

4 至 6 周后，如果您仍具有明显的抑郁症状，或

出现了曾以抗抑郁药物治疗的严重抑郁的征兆，

应请医生考虑使用抗抑郁药物。对抑郁的有效治

疗，可以让您的生活发生明显地改观。根据患者

描述，它就如同黑暗中的光明。有时，如果一种抗抑郁药不起作用，换用另一种可能会具有显著疗效。获知患者出现精神健康问题的精神病医生或家庭医生，有权开具抗抑郁处方药。

## WAY 26
## 方法 26

# BY TREATING ANY UNDERLYING BIPOLAR DISORDER WITH MEDICATIONS AND THERAPY

用药物和疗法治疗任何潜在躁郁症

Bipolar disorder is an illness in which the individual experiences dysfunctional ups and downs in their mood. These ups and downs are greater than the normal ups and downs of life. Such an altered mood states may last weeks or months. A milder form of this condition is called cyclothymic disorder. Such an individual may get trapped into using alcohol to deal with the fluctuating emotional states.

躁郁症是一种疾病。发病时，个体会经历机能失调性的个人情绪波动。与生活的正常起伏相比，这些情绪波动更为剧烈。这种变化的情绪状态，可能会持续数周或数月。更为温和的这种情绪波动被称为循环性精神疾病。这种人可能会酗酒，以此应对情绪波动。

If you or someone you know has such mood symptoms, you should obtain a psychiatric consult. The illness of bipolar disorder is serious but can be treated effectively with medications such as lithium or Depakote. Sobriety is much easier to achieve when the mood has been stabilized.

如果您或您认识的某人出现了这样的情绪症状，应该向精神病医生咨询。躁郁症是一种严重的疾病，但可以用诸如碳酸锂或丙戊酸钠这样的药物，进行有效治疗。情绪得到稳定后，戒酒就更容易实现了。

Some other clues about bipolar disorder are  the  symptoms of the mind going fast or experiencing   intense elation that lasts for several days. During   such states of elation, the energy level is increased,   libido and impulsivity are increased, and the need   for sleep  is decreased. A psychiatrist can help get   you on the right medication. The attainment of   sobriety along with treatment of bipolar disorder   will work synergistically, and the outlook for your   life can be dramatically better.

其他与躁郁症有关的提示性症状有：思维跳跃， 或经历持续数天的大喜、精力旺盛、性欲增强且 易冲动、睡眠需求减少。精神病医生可以帮助您 使用正确的药物。戒酒，与对躁郁症治疗的双管 齐下，会具有协同效果，极大地让您对未来充满希望。

# You can Do It 您可以做到

## WAY 27
## 方法 27

### BY TREATING ANY UNDERLYING ANXIETY PROBLEMS WITH MEDICATIONS AND THERAPY
用药物和疗法治疗任何潜在焦虑症

The treatment of anxiety with individual therapy was mentioned earlier. There are certain medications that can also be very effective in treating anxiety disorder.

用个体化疗法对焦虑症进行治疗，这是在较早前提出的。此外，某些药物也对焦虑症的治疗具有显著疗效。

If individual therapy alone is not enough, a combined approach using medications and therapy may be helpful.

如果单独运用个体化疗法疗效不够，药物与疗法双管齐下，或许会有帮助。

Some of the following medications have proven themselves as effective treatments for anxiety.

经证实，以下部分药物可以有效治疗焦虑症：

Paroxetine – This SSRI has a specific indication for social phobia. It is also effective for treatment of depression and anxiety related to other causes.

帕罗西汀-- 这种抗抑郁药明确适用于社交恐惧症。它还可以有效地治愈其他原因引起的抑郁与焦虑症。

Other SSRI medications marketed under brand names such as Zoloft, Celexa, Prozac, and others have all been found to be effective for treating anxiety syndromes. They take 3 to 6 weeks to achieve their effect. Patience therefore is the key.

市场出售的其他品牌抗抑郁药，如左洛复、百忧 解，及其他药物对治疗焦虑综合征的疗效均已被 发现。服用 3 至 6 周，就可以达到疗效。因 此， 耐心是关键。

Zoloft was one of the first medications to be approved for the treatment of PTSD (posttraumatic stress disorder). This problem is more common than is generally recognized.

左洛复是经批准，用于治疗创伤后精神紧张性精神障碍（创伤后应激障碍）的首选药物之一。这种病的普遍性，超越了人们的一般认知。

Buspirone (Buspar) has also been found to be effective for generalized anxiety. Benefits become noticeable in 2 to 3 weeks.

此外，已经发现丁螺环酮（布斯帕）对于一般性焦虑症的治疗是有效的。用药2至3周后，疗效显现。

Antihistamines such as hydroxyzine (Vistaril), have also been found to help with anxiety symptoms.

还发现抗组胺，如羟嗪（安太乐），能有助于缓解焦虑症状。

Benzodiazepines have also been effective for anxiety. There is some controversy about the use of benzodiazepines in individuals with alcoholism. The concern is that the benzodiazepines may trigger cravings for alcohol. In the individual that has a primary anxiety disorder, this risk may be less if benzodiazepines are used for a properly diagnosed anxiety disorder. Overall, it is probably better to try the other medications first for anxiety. If nothing else works, treatment of severe anxiety is safer with a benzodiazepine instead of the person trying to self- medicate with alcohol. Decisions for the use of benzodiazepines should be made on a case-by-case basis in consultation with the treating doctor. If benzodiazepines are used, alcohol should never be used concurrently. It can lead to respiratory suppression and death. Benzodiazepines by themselves are hardly ever lethal in overdose but may be lethal if combined with alcohol.

苯二氮平类药物也能有效治疗焦虑症。关于将这类药物用于酗酒者，还存在一些争议。争议的焦点在于，这类药物可能会触发酗酒者对饮酒的渴望。对于明显患有焦虑症的个体而言，如果将此类药物用于经正确诊断的焦虑症，这种风险可能更低。总之，首先尝试对焦虑症治疗有效的其他药物，或许会更好。如果都不起作用，用此类药物取代个体尝试以酗酒，对严重焦虑症进行的自我治疗，安全性更高。应该视具体情况，在咨询治疗医生的基础上，决定使用苯二氮平类药物。如果使用此类药物，则永远不要在用药期间饮酒。因为这会导致呼吸抑制及死亡。苯二氮平类药物本身的过量使用几乎是不致命的，但与酒精混合，则可能致命。

# WAY 28
方法 28

## BY TREATING ANY UNDERLYING ADHD
治疗任何潜在注意力不集中症

Individuals with ADHD show greater impulsivity and a propensity to get into trouble with alcohol use. Attention deficit hyperactivity disorder persists into adulthood in 30 to 40% of children that have ADHD. The prevalence of childhood ADHD is about 5 to 6% indicating that the condition is present in at least 2 to 3% of the adult population. Treatment of ADHD can be effective. There are various options for treatment including medications, various exercises and use of different strategies to anchor attention. The medications can help with impulsivity, and this can help to decrease the risks of alcoholism. The medications used to treat ADHD can either be a stimulant medication such as methylphenidate (Ritalin ER, Concerta), an amphetamine salt or combination (Adderall XR or Vyvanse) or a nonstimulant such as guanfacine (Intuniv), atomoxetine (Strattera), or clonidine. The use of stimulants for treatment of ADHD in adults should generally be avoided as there may be a higher risk of diversion and abuse. The nonstimulant medications have been found to equally effective and maybe safer. Providing treatment of ADHD can decrease risks of alcohol use disorder and many other complications related to ADHD. You may want to check out a book that I co-wrote with Professor Paramjeet Singh on ADHD. It is called Delivered from ADHD.

患有注意力不集中症(ADHD)的人表现出更为明显的冲动，并具有因饮酒招致麻烦的倾向。在患有 ADHD 的儿童中，注意缺陷多动障碍持续至成人期的比例为 30%至 40%。儿童 ADHD 患病率约为 5%至 6%，这表明目前患有该病的成人比例至少为 2%至 3%。可以对 ADHD 进行有效地治疗。可以选择的治疗方案多种多样，包括药物、各种锻炼，以及使用不同的办法，保持注意力集中。药物有助于缓解冲动，可以帮助降低酗酒的风险。用于治疗 ADHD 的药物，既可以是中枢神 经兴奋剂，如哌醋甲酯（利他林，哌甲酯制剂）、 苯丙胺盐，也可以是混合盐（苯丙胺混合盐或维 万斯），或非兴奋剂药物，如胍法辛（胍法新）、 阿托西汀（托莫西汀）或氯压定。通常，应避免 使用兴奋剂药物治疗成人 ADHD，因为药物滥用 的风险较高。 已经发现非兴奋剂药物对于成人 ADHD 具有同等的疗效，而且可能更加安全。对 ADHD 进行治疗，可以降低酗酒的风险，以及出 现其他与 ADHD 相关的多种并发症的风险。您或 许会希望查阅一本与 ADHD 相关的书籍，它是由 我与帕拉姆基特·辛格共同撰写完成的。本书链 接如下：

https://www.amazon.com/Delivered-ADHD- Overcoming-Children-Adults-ebook/dp/B00UDQU1SC/ref=sr_1_2?ie=UTF8&qid=1480659348&sr=8-2&keywords=Delivered+from+ADHD

## BY TREATING ANY ADJUSTMENT PROBLEMS

对任何适应症进行治疗

Psychiatrists and mental health professionals tend to minimize the role of adjustment disorders. Chronic conflicts at home or work can have a tremendous emotional impact. If these conflicts are resolved, dysfunctional coping by the use of alcohol or other drugs can be avoided. The risk for arguing, fighting and domestic violence at home is increased in the context of alcohol abuse. Use of alcohol may also lead to erratic behaviors at work and result in the loss of a job. Any act of aggression, drunk driving or other unlawful behaviors may lead to criminal charges and arrest. The way to overcome adjustment problems is to address the problems head on and separate out the factors that are under one's control and those that are not. This allows for the creation of an effective plan for overcoming the adjustment problems.

精神病医生及心理健康专家倾向于将适应症对人 造成的影响最小化。长期出现在家中，或工作场 所的冲突，可以对人的情绪造成巨大的影响。如 果冲突得到解决，就可以避免因酗酒或吸毒 而造成的机能性失调。滥饮，使争执、斗殴及家庭暴力的风险增加。酗酒还可能致使工作中行为古怪，而导致失业。任何侵犯行为、酒驾或其他非法行为，都可能招致获罪入狱。摆脱适应症的方法，就是要直面问题，并将产生因素按照可控与不可控进行区分，制定摆脱适应症的有效计划。

If you are having adjustment problems, you should seek individual therapy. Sometimes consultation with a priest or a wiser older person that you trust may be able to provide some answers for your situation.

如果您患有适应症，应该寻求个体化疗法。有时，就此咨询牧师或您所信任的更加睿智的长者，可能会让您获得解决问题的答案。

# WAY 30
# 方法 30

## BY BEING BORN AGAIN OR ADOPTING A STRONG RELIGIOUS FAITH

重新做人或拥有强烈的宗教信仰

If you are floundering in your faith, it may be time to look at different options that are out there. Many religions provide a close-knit community and offer support for a sober lifestyle. The matter of faith is a deeply personal one and should be made after deep introspection.

如果您没有固定的信仰，或许现在就是时候，了解其他不同的信仰了。许多教派都为信徒建立了关系亲密的社区，支持他们选择宁静的生活方式。信仰非常地个性化，应该在深刻的自我反省后确定。

You may want to consider some of the following religions that ban the use of alcohol.

您可能希望考虑以下一些教派，它们都禁酒：

- Amish and Quaker Christians are strict about prohibiting alcohol use. Pentecostals, Methodists, and Baptists in the Christian faith also believe that one should abstain from alcohol
  孟罗与贵格基督教严格禁酒。在基督教信仰中，五旬节派、循道公会教徒及浸礼宗教徒都认为不应该饮酒。

- Sikhism- Alcohol is forbidden for followers. There is an emphasis on a sober lifestyle, engaging in honest work and offering service to the community. There is a community of American Sikhs with a diverse website with meaningful information    at http://www.3ho.org/

锡克教—禁止信徒饮**酒**，注重适度饮酒的生活方式、诚实工作，为社区提供服务。有一个美国锡克教社区，开设了内容丰富的网站：http://www.3ho.org/，以此为大众提供有价值的信息。

- Buddhism, Jainism- The guidance is to walk the right path with an emphasis on a nonviolent and sober lifestyle.
  佛教、耆那教 — 引导信徒走正确的道路，强调没有暴力及适度饮酒的生活方式。

- The Church of Latter Day Saints prohibits alcohol and all other intoxicants.
  耶稣基督后期圣徒教会禁止饮酒及其他任何致醉物质的使用。

- Muslims- Abstinence from alcohol is almost universal.
  回教 — 几乎普遍禁酒。

- Hinduism, in general, emphasizes vegetarianism and a sober lifestyle.
  印度教 — 总体而言，印度教强调素食及适度饮酒的生活方式。

- Radha Soami faith has helped many to adopt a sober lifestyle through its focus on meditation and reflection.
  通过注重冥想与反思的罗陀香阿弥信仰，已经帮助许多人拥有了适度饮酒的生活方式。

There may be other sects and groups with spiritual leanings that prohibit alcohol.

或许还有其他的教派和群体，也具有禁酒的思想倾向。

As long as any of these faiths resonates with something inside you, you may decide to try out and follow one of these paths. It will help you stop alcohol use, and this may save your life.

只要任何信仰，与您的内心感受产生共鸣，就可以做出决定，摆脱现状，信奉其中一种。它会帮助您戒酒，而这可能会让您的生活得到拯救。

# You can Do It 您可以做到

## WAY 31
## 方法 31

### BY THE USE OF TOPAMAX TO ATTAIN SOBRIETY
用妥泰戒酒

Topiramate (Topamax) is an anticonvulsant agent that has shown some promise as an agent to decrease alcohol cravings. Individuals that were prescribed Topamax had an increase in the number of days that they were sober and decrease in the number of days of alcohol use.

托吡酯（妥泰）是一种抗惊厥制剂，已显示出作为一种降低酒精依赖制剂的初步成效。遵医嘱服用妥泰的酗酒者，适度饮酒天数增加，酗酒天数减少。

Like all other medications, the pros and cons should be discussed with your doctor.

与其他任何药物类似，应就使用本药的利弊，与医生进行讨论。

# WAY 32
## 方法 32

## BY USE OF LONG-ACTING NALTREXONE TO ATTAIN SOBRIETY

用长效纳曲酮戒酒

Naltrexone is an opiate antagonist that may help to decrease cravings for alcohol. This was mentioned earlier in the Sinclair method. This involved using the 50 mg tablet naltrexone tablet one hour every time before the planned use of alcohol. There are other ways of using naltrexone as well in the long-acting form. One of these is a long acting injection of naltrexone (Vivitrol) that can be given once a month. There is also a procedure to implant a naltrexone pellet that can release naltrexone slowly over a period of several months. They both can help with cutting down on cravings for alcohol if consistently used. Individuals with a certain opiate receptor gene variant may be more likely to benefit from naltrexone treatment. This is basically a fancy way of saying that if there is a family history of alcoholism; naltrexone may cut down that risk.

This long acting opiate blocker should not be used if there is a planned surgery scheduled in the near future. Due to the blockade of opiate receptors, the patient will not be able to get adequate pain relief from opiates that are often used in and around the time of surgery.

纳曲酮是一种阿片拮抗剂，可以帮助降低酒精依赖性。在之前的辛克莱尔法中，曾提到过该药。采用辛克莱尔法，需要在每次打算饮酒前的一小时，服用纳曲酮片剂 50 毫克。此外，还有其他以长效形式使用纳曲酮的方法。其中之一，就是每月注射一次长效纳曲酮（纳曲酮）。还有一种方法是将纳曲酮药丸放置体内，以便让药效在数月中缓慢释放。如果坚持使用，两

## You can Do It 您可以做到

种方法都能有助于降低人体对酒精的依赖性。出现某些麻醉剂受体基因变异的个体，或许从纳曲酮疗法中获得帮助的可能性更大。这基本上就等于说：如果个体具有酗酒家族史，纳曲酮就能降低其酗酒风险。如果近期计划安排外科手术，就不应使用这种长效麻醉阻断剂。因为麻醉剂受体的阻断，会让通常在手术期间及前后使用的麻醉剂，无法有效减轻病人的疼痛。

The use of an implant has been shown to increase the recovery rates for alcoholics that are trying to quit alcohol.

已经表明，纳曲酮体内放置法可以提高酗酒者的脱瘾康复率。

The implant can provide coverage for a period from 3 to 6 months.

体内放置法，可以让药效持续 3 至 6 个月。

More information can be found at the below website.
http://alcoholrehab.com/drug-addiction-treatment/naltrexone-implant-for-opiate-dependence/

登录以下网站，可获取更多信息：

  http://alcoholrehab.com/drug-addiction-treatment/naltrexone-implant-for-opiate-dependence/

## WAY33

## 方法 33

## WITH THE USE OF GABAPENTIN TO ATTAIN SOBRIETY

用加吧喷丁戒酒

Gabapentin has been used for the treatment of anxiety states. It may also offer a means of detoxing someone who has impaired liver function. A maintenance dose of gabapentin may help individuals along with PRN (as needed) naltrexone to overcome the cravings and to limit the dysfunctional use of alcohol. You should discuss this option with an addiction specialist to see if he has used this method. Most commonly, lorazepam and oxazepam are benzodiazepines that can also be used if liver function is compromised. The most damaging option, of course, is the continued use of alcohol.

加吧喷丁已被用于治疗焦虑症。对于肝功能已经受损的个体，它或许还是一种脱瘾方法。坚持服用加吧喷丁，并根据需要搭配服用纳曲酮，可以帮助个体摆脱酒瘾，并使酗酒造成的机能性失调得到抑制。您应该就此方案，与脱瘾专业人士进行讨论，了解他是否对其他病人用过该方法。大多数情况下，如果肝功能尚可，也可使用苯二氮平类药物氯羟去甲安定与去甲羟基安定脱瘾。当然，对人体肝功能的最大伤害，来自于持续饮酒

# WAY 34
## 方法 34

## BY THE USE OF ANTABUSE TO PREVENT RELAPSE TO ALCOHOL

用安塔布斯防止重新酗酒

Disulfiram (Antabuse) can help to limit the use of alcohol when a person is motivated but may waver in high risk situations. This medication stops the breakdown of alcohol and the intermediate product called acetaldehyde can cause very unpleasant symptoms. These include anxiety, nausea, vomiting and a rise in heart rate and respiratory rate. If the person has an underlying medical condition, it can get serious for them. The point of all this unpleasantness is of course to discourage the individual who is wavering in his resolve to not drink alcohol. If you are prescribed Antabuse, you are encouraged to never use alcohol, or take any medications that might have alcohol in it. Even dabbing yourself with an alcohol based cologne can trigger the Antabuse reaction in some people.

当人受到刺激，但又可能因饮酒带来的高风险而犹豫不决时，戒酒硫（安塔布斯）能发挥抑制作用。这种药物使被称为乙醛的酒精中间代谢产物降解受阻，造成人体极度不适，包括焦虑、恶心、呕吐、心跳加速及呼吸急促。如果个体患有潜在药物过敏，这会让其不适加剧。关键在于，所有这些不适，对于还没有决心戒酒的人而言，理所当然地起到了促进他们戒酒的作用。如果医生为您开具了处方药安塔布斯，建议您不要饮酒，或服用可能含有酒精的任何药物。在部分人员中，即便涂抹以酒精为基质的古龙香水，也会引发安塔布斯反应。

## WAY 35
## 方法 35

### BY RECOGNIZING THE DIFFERENT FACTORS ASSOCIATED WITH ALCOHOLISM- AND AVOIDING USE OF ALCOHOL

认识到与酗酒及避免饮酒有关的不同因素

There are many factors that contribute to alcoholism. Genetics however seem to account for about 50% of the risk. This is very significant and a strong reason for those with alcoholism in their family member to never take to drinking. One of the genes implicated has been the opiate receptor gene Asp40. Other genes have also been implicated. For now the only indicator of a genetic risk is the family history. In the near future however, we should be able to cheaply determine all the genes that place us at risk for various diseases. If we have a particular vulnerability for an illness such as heart disease, a certain cancer or alcoholism, we can take steps to limit exposure to circumstances that increase the risk for developing that disease.

造成酗酒的因素多种多样。不过，似乎有 50%的风险来源于遗传。对于有家庭成员酗酒的个体而言，要做到从不饮酒，遗传因素会起到非常关键且突出的作用。牵涉其中的一种基因，是麻醉受体基因 Asp40。其他基因也具有相关性。就目前而言，提示存在基因风险的唯一指征，就是家族酗酒史。但在不远的将来，我们应该能够方便地检测出将人类置于各种疾病风险中的所有基因。如果出现了某些疾病的特定易损性，如心脏病、某种癌症或酗酒，我们可以采取步骤，限制自己接触到能增加该病患病风险的环境。

In the case of alcoholism, if we find that there is a risk from our genetic profile, we can almost mark alcohol as an allergy is order to abstain from it for a lifetime. It is almost as serious as being allergic to penicillin. Exposure to the both is deadly if you are vulnerable.

至于酗酒，如果我们发现有基因风险，完全可以将酒精作为一种过敏源，终生戒酒。酒精过敏的严重性，几乎等同于盘尼西林过敏。如果您是易受损者，那么，接触这两种物质都是致命的。

The below diagram is a convoluted way of representing the risk. The big circle at the center represents the genetic risk. The little intersecting circles represent various factors that increase the risk. Exposure to alcohol is like throwing a lighted match into a tinder box if some of these risk factors are present. Avoiding exposure to alcohol if you have some of the below risk factors is the key to avoiding troubles.

下面的图表稍显复杂，它对这种风险进行了描绘。中心大圈代表基因风险，相交的小圈代表增加风险的各种因素。如果这些风险因素中的部分出现，饮酒就犹如向易燃物中扔进一根点燃的火柴。如果您有以下部分风险因素，避免饮酒，这是不发生问题的关键。

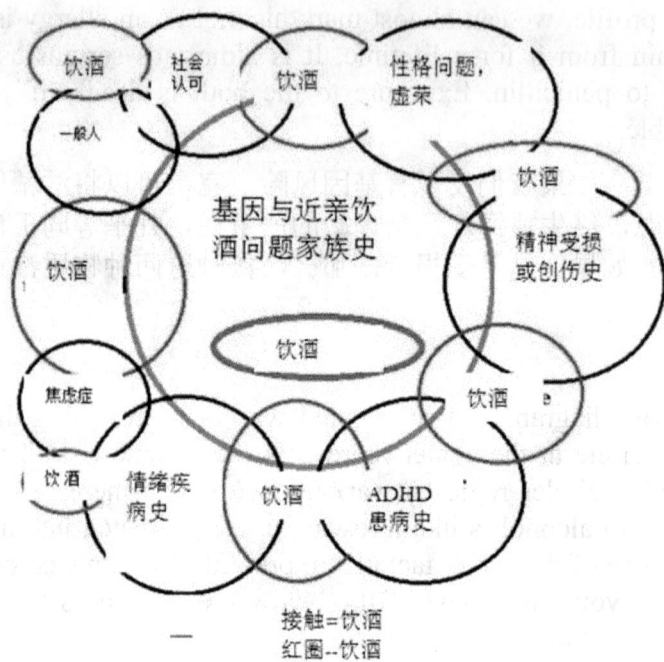

饮酒
社会认可
饮酒
性格问题，虚荣
一般人
饮酒
精神受损或创伤史
基因与近亲饮酒问题家族史
饮酒
饮酒
焦虑症
饮酒
饮酒
情绪疾病史
饮酒
ADHD患病史

接触=饮酒
红圈--饮酒

# WAY 36
## 方法 36

## BY RECOGNIZING THAT ALCOHOLISM IS SIMILAR TO THE CARNIVOROUS PITCHER PLANT
认识到酗酒与食肉猪笼草的相似之处

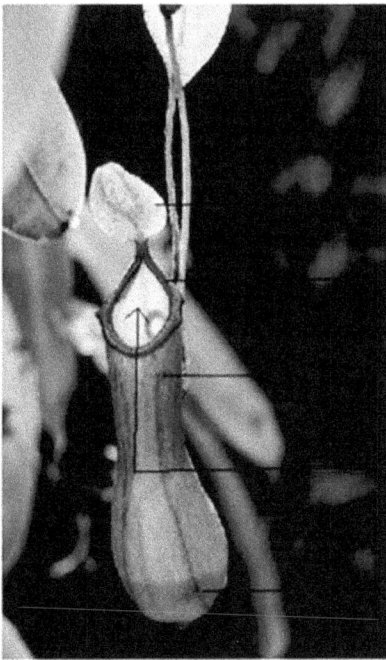

美丽的翼瓣

分布在边缘的花蜜

芬芳的香味

杯状内层巨大的斜度

正垂死挣扎的、看不见的猎物

*Advertisement*

猪笼草与酗酒，都是致命的陷阱

Alcohol is comparable to the carnivorous pitcher plant. It's vibrant colors and glossy leaves attract insects flying by. The curious insect lands and unaware of the trap, begins to drink the sticky sweet sap on the surface of the pitcher plant. Soon however, it finds itself weighed down and is unable take off. The wings have also gotten sticky in the meantime from the sap. As the insect slides downward, the slope of the pitcher plant surface becomes more and more steep and then impossible. The poor hapless insect does not have a prayer as it dangles and falls to its death in the cauldron of digestive juices at the bottom of the pitcher like stomach of the plant.

可以把酗酒比作食肉猪笼草。猪笼草斑斓而闪亮的叶片，吸引了从它身边飞过的昆虫。好奇的昆虫停在花瓣上，丝毫没有意识到这是一个陷阱，开始吸吮猪笼草表面既粘又甜的树液。但不久，它发现自己变重了，飞不起来了，翅膀也同时被树液黏住了。随着昆虫滑入猪笼草内侧，其内侧面的坡度越来越陡，然后昆虫完全失去了脱身的可能。可怜而倒霉的昆虫连一个祷告者也没有，就摇摇晃晃地掉下去，死在了类似植物胃部、猪笼草底部的那一腔消化液中。

Alcohol is similar in many of its ways.

在许多方面，酗酒与此类似。

It lures as well through glitzy ads. It promises a good time, and soon weighs down the person with clumsiness of intoxication and later with a hangover and depression. A persons' body over a short period will need more and more just to feel normal – the slope is changing. The symptoms of withdrawal lead to a need to continue drinking. This vicious cycle leads to a steep decline in emotional and physical health- the slope has gotten even steeper. Over time, it gets worse at an even faster rate as part of the liver dies and gets replaced by scar tissue (cirrhosis). In this cauldron are added accidents, divorce, and arrests among others- the slope has become impossible.

借助炫目的广告，酒也对人充满了诱惑。它承诺为您带来了一段美好的时光，却在稍后，让人陷入过量饮酒的愚钝，以及再后来的宿醉与抑郁之中。短时间后，人体会越来越需要感觉正常— 犹如昆虫感觉到坡度正在变化。停止饮酒的不适，导致了继续饮酒需求的产生。这种恶性循环会带来情绪及心理健康的极具下降—犹如坡度变得越来越陡。一段时间后，随着部分肝脏功能的丧失，以及被疤痕组织取代（肝硬化），人体健康状况更快速地恶化。此外，再加之意外事故、离婚以及获刑— 这个人就不可能死里逃生了。

As these problems mount, the individual is increasingly trapped into a state of no return. The individual may have many medical maladies, remains confused from the elevated liver ammonia that his or liver cannot handle. The end is always rapid and unexpected due to any number of different complications that can arise in this fragile medical state. Alcohol in short has done what the pitcher plant did to the hapless insect.

伴随这些问题的增加，个体日益陷入无力自拔的境地。他可能还有一些医学疾病，依然对自己或肝脏无法应对的肝氨升高不明就里。但这个阶段的病人很脆弱，不同并发症发生一种或多种，都总会使结果迅速而又出人意料的出现。简而言之，饮酒的作用，就等同于猪笼草对倒霉昆虫所做的一切。

You should always keep the picture of the dead  insects in the pitcher plant in mind when thinking of alcohol. Do not be fooled by the false advertisements promised on the TV and the billboards.

当您想饮酒时，应该想到这张猪笼草里死去昆虫的照片。不要受电视和广告牌上，那些做出承诺的虚假广告的愚弄。

If you are at high risk, alcohol can ensnare and create these significant problems in your life if you give it half a chance.

如果您在高风险中，并具有 50%的酗酒机会，那么，饮酒会让您上瘾，并为您的生活带来严重的问题。

The pitcher plant and alcohol are both unforgiving and both exact the ultimate price.

猪笼草和酗酒的危害都是不可原谅的，也都会让人付出最大的代价。

## WAY 37
## 方法 37

### RELIGIOUS PILGRIMAGE , FINDING ROOTS AS A TREATMENT

宗教朝圣之旅，把找到个体的本源作为治疗方法

Some individuals after a successful detox may benefit from going on a religious pilgrimage or some tour of self-discovery back to their roots. Many individuals that are on a religious pilgrimage feel a calling to improve their lives and experience a quickening of their religious zeal. This can help to curb the instinct to use alcohol. When one is serious about making a real change, a pilgrimage may support and bolster the plan for recovery. It will provide the emotional and religious support that one needs during the early phases when cravings can arise. If the doctor has provided any medications, these should be taken as prescribed. There should be a backup plan if there is a relapse or if there are any complications. Antabuse may help to bolster sobriety efforts at times of increased relapse risk or cravings. Travel with a friend or family member is helpful as they can offer additional support as needed.

成功脱瘾后的一些人，可能因一次宗教朝圣之旅，或回到其本源的自我发现之旅而得到帮助。正在朝圣之旅中的许多人，感受到一种提升自己生活的内心召唤，经历了自身宗教热情的一种复苏。这有助于抑制饮酒的冲动。当一个人认真做出真正改变时，朝圣或许对其脱瘾康复计划具有支持与支撑作用。在会产生酒精依赖的早期阶段，朝圣会为个体提供所需的情感及宗教支持。如果医生开具了任何药物，应该按处方服用。如果出现重新饮酒，或出现任何并发症，应备份有解决方案。在复饮或酒精依赖风险上升时，安塔布斯可能会有助于戒酒。与朋友

或家人结伴旅行，是对此有帮助的，因为他们可以提供所需的
其他支持。

## WAY 38
## 方法 38

### BY LIVING IN AN AREA WHERE ALCOHOL IS BANNED
迁居禁酒地区

If you are planning to consolidate your recovery and need extra help, it may be worthwhile moving to an area where alcohol is not sold for religious or other policy reasons. There are some areas in the world where alcohol is banned by the government as they feel it is too much of a risk for a large number of people. Such a place can be a haven for if you have struggled with alcohol problems. You may even consider taking a job there to consolidate your recovery. Countries that ban the sale of liquor are listed alphabetically below.

如果您正计划巩固脱瘾康复，并需要进一步地帮助，迁居因为宗教或其他政治原因，而不出售酒的地区，可能是有意义的。世界上有一些地区的政府禁止饮酒，因为他们认为饮酒对于大部分民众而言，风险太大。如果您正因酗酒而焦头烂额，这种地区堪称绝佳的选择。您甚至可以考虑在这里工作，以便对自己的脱瘾康复进行巩固。禁止售酒的国家按字母顺序排列如下：

Afghanistan ,Bangladesh, Brunei, INDIA (In certain parts such as Gujarat, Mizoram, Manipur, Nagaland and Lakshadweep) Iran Kuwait Libya,Saudi Arabia,Sudan UAE,Yemen ,Pakistan.

阿富汗、孟加拉、文莱

印度（部分地区，如古吉拉特邦、米佐拉姆邦、曼尼普尔、那加兰邦及洛克沙维）

伊朗、科威特、利比亚、沙特阿拉伯、苏丹

# Overcoming Alcohol 摆脱酗酒

阿联酋、也门、巴基斯坦

Some of these countries are embroiled in violence and not exactly prime locations for a safe neighborhood. As an alternative, there may be communities where you live that are sober. If there is a locality or neighborhood that are teetotalers, you should seek to live there if sobriety is important for you. Going to a church where sobriety is an article of faith provides a readymade community for those seeking to lead a sober and healthy life. You can also create your own sober circle by only socializing with friends that are also committed to sobriety. It is worth the effort that it might take. Soon, you may find that it is the only way to live a rich and fulfilling life.

其中的一些国家正陷入暴力冲突之中，的确不是 找到可靠邻居的首选之地。取而代之，您也可以 迁居到主张适度饮酒的社区生活。如果有一个地 方禁酒，或周围的人都是禁酒主义者，而禁酒对 您而言又非常重要，那么，您应该设法去那里生 活。在教会，禁酒是信仰的一部分。因此，参 加教会可以为那些寻求适度饮酒健康生活的人士， 提供一个现成的社区。您还可以只与也希望戒酒的朋友交往，创建自己的戒酒群体。这种努力可能会发挥作用，所以是值得为之的。不久，您会发现这是让自己过上富足、充实生活的唯一途径

。

## WAY 39
### 方法 39

## BY USING ACAMPROSATE (CAMPRAL)

用阿坎酸（阿坎酸）戒酒

This medication has been used by some people to curb cravings for alcohol. When combined with other treatments such as group therapy, it can be helpful. The most common side effect is diarrhea. It should not be used by those with impaired kidney function. You should check with your doctor to see if this is a good option for you.

已有一些人用这种药抑制酒精依赖性。与其他治疗方法，如群体疗法，合并使用时，该药会功效显著。其最常见的副作用是造成腹泻。肾功能受损的人，不应使用该药。应咨询医生，了解该药是否是适合自己的最佳选择。

# WAY 40
## 方法 40

## SIMPLE COUNSELING BY A DOCTOR CAN HELP DECREASE ALCOHOL USE

医生的简单建议，可以帮助您减少饮酒量

Sometimes, your doctor may comment on your abnormal laboratory tests that could be related to alcohol use. The doctor can also administer simple questionnaires such as the CAGE questionnaire to see if you have a problem with alcohol. CAGE stands for the following:

有时，针对您可能与饮酒相关的化验数据异常，医生可以提供意见。此外，他们还可以通过简单的问卷调查，比如 CAGE 问卷调差，了解您是否酗酒。CAGE 含义如下：

C- stands for if you have tried to cut down on alcohol on your own

代表您是否尝试依靠自己戒酒；

A Stands for if you have been annoyed by someone telling you that you may be drinking too much.

代表您是否因他人说您可能过量饮酒而懊恼；

G-Stands for if you feel guilty about how much you drink

代表您是否为自己的饮酒量而感到内疚；

tands for if you have taken an eye opener in the mornings to steady your nerves from the morning withdrawal symptoms.

代表您是否在早晨有停止饮酒症状，为了稳定紧张情绪而出现异常。

If the answer is a yes to two or more of these questions, the doctor should ask you further about your alcohol use habits. The doctor can then counsel you to cut back and also offer other treatment options that are available in the community. Studies have shown that this type of counseling does make a difference in the long run.

如果针对其中两项或更多项的答案是肯定的，那么，医生应进一步了解您的饮酒习惯。随后，他会建议您减少饮酒，还会为您提供社区现有的其他治疗方法。研究表明，就长期而言，这类咨询意义重大。

Modern-day doctors are well trained to recognize alcohol-related problems.

当今的医生们，都接受过系统的培训，可以识别与酗酒相关的问题。

## WAY 41
## 方法 41

## BY INTERVENTION AFTER AN ACCIDENT
意外事故后介入

If there is an accident as a result of alcohol, the person may have to be taken to the emergency room. Once the immediate health care needs are met, counseling by a doctor about alcohol treatment options can be helpful. The doctor will make an assessment of any withdrawal symptoms. He will review any detoxification needs and may offer the treatment options to you. Interventions at moments of such crisis in the emergency room can sometimes make a big difference.

如果发生了酗酒导致的意外事故，个体可能不得不被送入急诊室。得到紧急救治后，立即就戒酒治疗的方案与医生进行咨询，会非常有用。医生会评估任何的停止饮酒症状，审度脱瘾治疗的任何需求，还可能为您提供脱瘾治疗的多种方案。在急救室的这种危机时刻，介入脱瘾治疗，有时会非常有效。

Sometimes alcohol and addiction counselors are available and can be asked to meet with you by the doctor.

有时，急诊室配备有酗酒与上瘾咨询人员，可以要求他们陪同您与医生进行商讨。

Such counselling in the emergency room can take on an added poignancy because of the events that have just occurred. It is one of the ways that      some individuals receive help. They are able to come to terms with their problems and begin their road to recovery. Whatever opportunity works to help the individual should be utilized. If you are the individual in the emergency room with the alcohol problem, recognize that you are luck you are still alive. Do take this opportunity to straighten out your life and start the process of recovery and healing. There may be legal charges sometimes that you will have to contend with. Your commitment to sobriety will help you in getting a better disposition by a judge. Work with  your attorney and your counselors to do  what  you need  to  do. You should  be  honest  in  your  intentions  however. Falsehood will not fool anyone.

急诊室的这种咨询，可以因为已经发生的意外，而变得更加尖锐。但这是一些人接受帮助的其中一种方式。他们可以因此承认自己的问题，并开始步入康复。无论任何机会，只要能发挥作用，为个体提供帮助，就应该采用。如果现在您就因酗酒而身处急救室，要认识到自己是幸运的，因为您还活着。好好利用这次机会，让自己的生活发生改变，开始康复过程，并让自己痊愈。有时，您可能不得不面对法庭指控。承诺戒酒，会帮助您获得法官的轻判。与律师和咨询人员合作，履行您需要承担的责任。但您应诚实说出自己的意图，因为谎言愚弄不了所有的人。

## WAY 42
## 方法 42

## BY GETTING HELP IN JAIL OR PRISON
让拘留所或监狱帮您戒酒

Domestic violence is often related to alcohol use in some families. The perpetrator may end up in jail. Here, an assessment is made of any alcohol and substance abuse problems such as dependence. If you drink on a regular basis and end up in the slammer, you should let the nurse on duty know so that withdrawal complications from alcohol can be prevented. She or he will also ask you about other conditions, and it is important to be truthful.

通常，出现在一些家庭中的家暴与饮酒有关。施暴者可能会被关进拘留所。这里会对他们的任何酒精及物质滥用问题，如酒精依赖性做出评估。如果您每天饮酒，那么，在这里将无法饮酒。因此，您应就停止饮酒的并发症，提醒值班护士，以防止出现任何并发症。值班护士还会问及您的其他情况，如实回答，这非常重要。

# You can Do It 您可以做到

## WAY 43
## 方法 43

### STIPULATION BY CHILD PROTECTIVE SERVICES (CPS) FOR A PARENT TO GET HELP FOR THEIR ALCOHOL AND DRUG RELATED PROBLEMS

按照儿童保护服务条款对家长的要求，

获得对酗酒及吸毒有关问题的帮助

Unfortunately, this is another way that individuals can get backed into getting help for themselves that they may have otherwise delayed. The resulting event is often charges of possible child neglect or abuse due to the children being unkempt, not attending school or wandering away from home. The child protective services may go into the home and find drug use paraphernalia, extreme disorganization and filth indicating that alcohol or drug use is impairing the parents. Many parents have been trapped into the cycle of addiction are unable to get out of the trap. If you find yourself in this situation, look at the silver lining and try to take advantage of the treatment program offered to you.

遗憾的是，这可能是被个体延误的另一种方法，但它可以重新让其获得帮助。违反儿童保护服务条款，通常会导致各种指控，包括因儿童举止粗野、不想上学或离家出走，而可能对忽视或虐待儿童。儿童保护服务机构人员可能会进入房间，找出吸毒用具，发现房间内的脏乱不堪，这表明酗酒或吸毒正在削弱父母承担子女责任的能力。许多家长已经陷入成瘾的恶性循环中，无力自拔。如果您发现自己处于这种状况下，要心怀希望，努力利用得到的治疗计划。

# WAY 44
## 方法 44

## BY FILLING UP YOUR SCHEDULE
让自己忙起来

They say that an empty mind is a devil's workshop. There is some truth to this. A sense of emptiness and boredom may become precursors to drinking. To combat this, one should fill up the schedule so that it is filled with the pursuit of hobbies, special interests or and volunteer activities where you may be able to help others. This will avoid the feelings of emptiness and boredom. Scheduling a meaningful day with enough periods of rest can be the cornerstone of all recovery efforts for some people. Happiness and contentment are too important to leave to chance.

人们都说，空空如也的大脑是魔鬼出没之地。一定程度而言，这是个事实。感觉空虚和无聊，可能导致酗酒。为了战胜这种感觉，应该让自己忙起来，追求自己的爱好、特殊兴趣，或从事可以为其他人提供帮助的自愿者活动，以此将自己的时间填满，避免空虚与无聊。让自己休息充足，度过有意义的每一天，充足地休息，可以成为部分人所有康复努力的转折点。快乐与满足都太重要，不要听天由命。

This can be planned for, and scheduling activities to fill enough of your schedule is a part of this recovery effort.

对自己的日程进行规划，安排活动将它填满，这是康复努力的一部分。

You can Do It 您可以做到

# WAY 45
# 方法 45

## BY RECOGNIZING BY THE PREGNANT WOMAN THAT SHE IS RESPONSIBLE FOR ANOTHER LIFE AND DECIDING TO QUIT

孕妇要认识到自己对另一个生命的责任而决心

戒酒

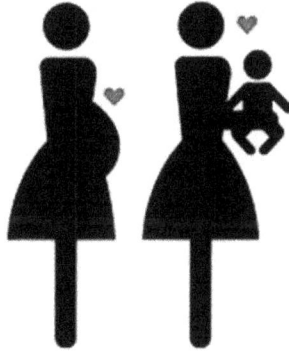

A woman can be educated about the fact that no amount of alcohol is safe for the baby. Some wine industry sponsored studies have tried to create guidelines for safe drinking by pregnant mothers. This irrationality can only be explained by greed that drives these sponsered studies. The child can be permanently harmed with various facial feature deformities and mental retardation. Smaller amounts of alcohol still do damage. The syndrome has been well recognized and is called Fetal Alcohol Syndrome. If you google this, you will find pictures of these children damaged by alcohol. Some of the direct effects from fetal alcohol exposure include brain damage leading to a small head (microcephaly) along with an arrested development of various facial features.

女性要接受一个事实：对于胎儿而言，任何饮酒量都是不安全的。一些酒厂提供赞助，尝试研究创建孕妇安全饮酒指南。对这种不理性行为的唯一解释就是：贪婪促使这些研究得到赞助。孕妇饮酒，会让儿童永久地受到伤害，出现各种面部特征畸形及智力缺陷。再小的饮酒量，都会对胎儿造成伤害。这种综合征已经得到了充分地认识，被称为胎儿酒精综合征。如果用谷歌搜索这种病症，您会找到受酒精损伤的婴儿图片。接触酒精对胎儿造成的直接影响包括大脑损伤，这会导致小头症（头小畸形），以及各种面部特征发育停滞。

# You can Do It 您可以做到

## WAY 46
## 方法 46

### OVERCOMING ALCOHOL WITH THE THREE P'S: PATIENCE, PERSISTENCE AND PERSEVERANCE
### 摆脱酗酒三原则：耐心、恒心与毅力

In combating alcohol-related problems, you will have to be both patient and persistent in your efforts. It is not unknown to have a slip-up or a relapse. The key is to get back up, dust yourself off and to persevere with persistence. With continued efforts, alcohol becomes a distant memory, and your roots will grow strong in sobriety and your new found lifestyle. This does not mean that one can become complacent, however.

在与酗酒的抗衡过程中，您必须要努力付出耐心 与恒心。出现失误或反弹，这是尽人皆知的。关 键是要重振旗鼓，打起精神，凭借恒心坚持到底。 通过不断地努力，酗酒会成为您遥远的记忆，您 会从根本上更加坚定地戒酒，并找到自己全新的 生活方式。但这不意味着您会变得骄傲自满。

One need to avoid follow the treatment plan and use the strategies that have worked before. A simple strategy amongst others is to always have the number of your sponsor or key friend or family member on speed dial so that you can summon help for the periods when you are feeling stressed and need to talk.

一个人需要避免对治疗计划的盲从，而应使用之 前有效的戒酒方法。始终保留您的支持者、挚友或家庭成员的快速拨号方式，以便在感觉压力并需要交流时能求助，这是其中一种简单的方法。

# Overcoming Alcohol 摆脱酗酒

# You can Do It 您可以做到

## WAY 47
## 方法 47

### INTERVENTION- FRIENDS AND LOVED ONES AS A GROUP ASK THE ALCOHOLIC TO GET HELP
### 介入--朋友和爱人共同要求酗酒者寻求帮助

This process is called an intervention. In this strategy, the family and friends of the alcoholic gather together for a meeting with the alcoholic. They talk to the alcoholic one at a time about how their alcoholism is affecting them. If you are part of this group, it is ok to write out what you are going to say before you say it. These concerned people then ask the alcoholic as a group to agree to get help for drinking. The alcoholic will often agree. At this point, an arrangement should already have been made in consultation with a treatment specialist for an inpatient admission for detox and further rehabilitation.

这个过程被称为介入性治疗。使用这种方法，酗酒者的家人和朋友一起，与酗酒者见面，和盘托出酗酒对他们造成影响的程度。如果您身为朋友或爱人，最好在交谈前写下要说的话。随后，相关的人员会作为一个整体，要求酗酒者同意获取戒酒帮助。通常，酗酒者会同意这个要求。这时，适合同意脱瘾及进一步康复患者的戒酒计划应该已经制定完成，且该计划的制定咨询过治疗专业人士。

# WAY 48
# 方法 48

## MARITAL AND COUPLE COUNSELLING CAN HELP
### 婚姻辅导及夫妻咨询有助于戒酒

The problem of marital strife in the life of the alcoholic is often underestimated when making plans for recovery. Marital and couples counseling can help to heal and repair past emotional injuries and insults. This can be immensely important in the overall recovery process. Settling some of these conflicts and misunderstandings between couples can decrease the anxiety surrounding such conflicts. This can lessen the urge for the use of alcohol. The individual with the alcohol problem will more readily go into detox, and this counseling can continue through the recovery and maintenance phase. The best therapy occurs when both have achieved sobriety. Having a partner who understands can be a tremendous gift when trying to overcome alcohol.

制定脱瘾康复计划时，酗酒对婚姻生活不和谐的影响，常常被低估。婚姻辅导及夫妻咨询有助于治愈并修复曾经的情感创伤与伤害。在整个康复过程中，这一点非常重要。其中一些冲突的平息和误解的消除，可以减少这些冲突所带来的焦虑，让饮酒的冲动降低。这种咨询会让酗酒者更乐意接受脱瘾治疗，并在康复和维持期继续进行咨询。当夫妻双方都成功戒酒时，最佳疗效出现。在您设法摆脱酗酒时，有一个善解人意的伴侣陪伴左右，这是一种莫大的恩赐。

You can Do It 您可以做到

## WAY 49
### 方法 49

## MOTIVATIONAL ENHANCEMENT THERAPY
动机强化疗法

This is a popular therapy for alcoholism and other addictions. It can help as it meets the person where they are at. It does not condemn but merely helps the individual examine his or her life situation and helps in examining the options that may be available for recovery. It invites and encourages the individual to look at the pros and cons of their drinking objectively. They are encouraged to take logical steps based on their self-analysis.

这是一种常用疗法，适用于酗酒及其他成瘾者。 对于适应这种疗法的人而言，它能发挥作用。该疗法只是帮助个体审视自己的生活状况，以及对可能有助于脱瘾康复的多种选择做出验证，而不指责个体。它带领并鼓励个体客观地看待酗酒的利与弊。受到鼓励的酗酒者，会在自我分析的基础上，采取合理的步骤脱瘾。

# WAY 50
## 方法 50

## BY GIVING UP OF HUBRIS AND EXCESSIVE PRIDE
摒弃傲慢与过分骄傲

In Proverbs 16:18, it is stated that "Pride goes before destruction and a haughty spirit before stumbling."

箴言篇第 16 章 18 行说"骄傲导致毁灭，自大铸成大错。"

Hubris is haughty and excessive pride. If this is in in the character makeup of the alcoholic, it becomes difficult to offer help to him or her.

傲慢等于自大与过分骄傲。如果酗酒者的性格中包含这两点，要帮助他脱瘾就会困难重重。

This toxic pride causes the person to deny their problem even it is obvious that their life is in shambles due to alcohol. Any admission of a problem is a knock on their sense of being perfect. They are used to being in control.

骄傲有害，会让酗酒者否认自己的问题，即便生活因酗酒而一片混乱是显而易见的。对问题的任何承认，都会对他们保持完美的感觉形成冲击。他们习惯于控制一切。

If you are such a person, you can learn to give up the need for excessive perfection and pride. You can show you are stronger by admitting that you have a problem.

如果您是这样的人，要学会放弃对过分完美与骄傲的需求。承认问题，您可以展示出自己的更加强大。

Once you can give up the excessive pride, you can accept the first tenet of recovery, an admission that we were powerless over alcohol and needed help. It is in humility that your salvation lies. Humility allows us to adopt a new lifestyle of sobriety. Once you accept that you need help, you are already there.

只要能放弃过分骄傲，您就能接受脱瘾康复这条第一原则，承认自己曾对酗酒无能为力，并需要帮助。谦逊，让您获得拯救。谦逊让您得以过上戒酒的全新生活方式。只要您认可自己需要帮助，就已经得到帮助了。

The next step is to get detoxed in a supervised setting that is most convenient. After this, you can explore other treatment options with your doctor and treatment team. You can perhaps can take the message of redemption to others who are also Struggling.

下一步，就是要在监护下脱瘾，这是最容易的。此后，您可以与医生及治疗团队，摸索其他的治疗方法。或许，您还可以把自己得救的经历，与还在为脱瘾而挣扎的其他人分享。

## BONUS CHAPTER
### 奖励篇

### 1. ANTISMOKING DRUG FOR ALCOHOL
适用于戒酒的戒烟药

There is some evidence that the antismoking drug Varenicline can decrease cravings for alcohol. An addiction specialist can discuss the pros and cons of this agent. Some serious effects on mood in a minority of patients have been noted, and these need to be taken into consideration.

有证据表明，戒烟药伐尼克兰可以使酒瘾减弱。成瘾专业人士能够阐明这种制剂的利与弊。需要注意的是，这种药会对少数患者的情绪造成严重影响。因此，要将这些需求纳入考虑之中。

### 2 NUTRITIONAL DEFICIENCIES
营养不良

Nutritional deficiencies commonly exist in those with alcohol use disorders. Some of The common deficiencies associated with alcoholism include deficiencies of folic acid, vitamin B12, selenium, zinc, various other B- complex vitamins, vitamin C, vitamin A, Vitamin D, and deficiencies of l-carnitine, and other micronutrients. Some believe that by providingmicronutrient supplementation, withdrawal may be better managed, and recovery from mood symptoms may be accelerated. It would make sense since these micronutrients are intimately involved in many neurological functions.

**You can Do It 您可以做到**

患有酒精使用障碍的人，通常营养不良。与酗酒相关的一般营养不良，包括叶酸、维生素 B12、硒元素、锌元素、其他各种 B 型复合维生素、维生素 C、维生素 A、维生素 D 缺乏，以及 L-肉碱及其他微量营养物质的不足。一些人认为，通过补充微量营养物质，可能更有效地戒酒，也能更快地让情绪症状得到康复。这种说法    可能不无道理，因为这些微量营养物质与部    分神经系统功能密切相关。

# MORE ABOUT INPATIENT AND OUTPATIENT DETOXES

## AN INPATIENT DETOX

住院脱瘾与门诊脱瘾补充说明

This is the way that most detoxes are conducted. Once the individual makes a decision to detox and quit, his family or friends can help him or her get ready for this. This will include obtaining leave from work and gathering insurance information and any extra funds that may be needed to accomplish the detox.

住院脱瘾与门诊脱瘾，这是绝大部分脱瘾诊所都采用的脱瘾方法。酗酒者一旦决定脱瘾及戒酒，家人或朋友就可以帮助他们为此做好准备，包括向单位请假、收集保险资料，以及完成脱瘾可能需要的任何其他基金的资料。

A person should be driven to the detox facility to avoid last minute change of plans. The family and friends can provide collateral information to the doctors and nurses when they do the initial interview and intake.

应促使酗酒者到脱瘾机构接受脱瘾治疗，避免其临时改变计划。在医生和护士首次与酗酒者的家人和朋友谈话并了解情况时，家人和朋友可以向他们提供酗酒者的间接信息。

If you are the one being admitted, you will be given a physical exam after the initial history along with the common laboratory workup to rule out any major medical problems or concerns. The laboratory workup may include tests such as the comprehensive metabolic profile [CMP], the complete blood count [CBC], a thyroid profile and a urinalysis. Some doctors may order a carbohydrate deficient transferrin test or the %CDT. The % CDT is marker to test for heavy use of alcohol (more than 5 drinks in men and more than 4 in women) over the last 2 weeks. Once the patient is admitted, the vital signs of the patient may be monitored every 2 or every 4 hours. The patient is placed on a 4 to a 5-day tapering dose of a suitable benzodiazepine. Thiamine, multivitamins, folic acid, are also ordered. Additional PRN (as needed) benzodiazepines are used to control breakthrough alcohol withdrawal symptoms. Sometimes magnesium sulfate is given as an injection to lower the risk of tremors and convulsions. The person is provided nutritious, balanced meals although the appetite may not be great for the first two days of withdrawal. Any nausea is treated by adequate control of withdrawal symptoms. Antinausea medications are rarely needed. A doctor usually makes rounds every day. On the fourth day, most of the withdrawal symptoms begin to subside, and subsequent plans are made for enrollment in groups for your further recovery. A 30-day program is usually offered, but shorter inpatient stays are also effective.

如果您是接受脱瘾治疗的人，会在病史询问及常规化验后，按要求进行体检，以便排除任何重大疾病或健康问题。化验可能包括各种检测，如全面的新城代谢图谱[CMP]、完整血项[CBC]、甲状腺情况及验尿。有些医生可能还会要求做碳水化合物缺乏转移检测或糖缺失性转铁蛋白百分比检查。这项指标是为了检测病人在近两周的过量（男性超过5次，女性超过4次）饮酒情况。患者一旦入院，医院会每天监测其生命体征2或4小时，并依照安排，在4至5天的时间里，以递减剂量服用苯二氮平类药物。此外，还会按要求服用硫胺素、复合维生素及叶酸。按需添加的苯二氮平类药物用于控制停止饮酒症状的突然出现。有时，会为其注射硫酸镁，降低出现颤抖与抽搐的风险。尽管在停止饮酒的最初1至2天，患者进食量可能不大，但还是要进食营养物质，平衡膳食供应。任何的恶心都可以通过充分控制停止饮酒症状得到治疗，很少使用止吐剂。通常，医生会每天查房。入院第四天，绝大部分停止饮酒症状开始消退，可以制定您进一步参与群体脱瘾康复的后续计划了。

通常的住院脱瘾计划为期 30 天，但略短与此的天数也不会对疗效有影响。

Before discharge, an outpatient treatment plan is developed that may involve attending various self- groups such as AA or secular groups in the community. Therapist led groups are also recommended.

出院前，要制定好门诊治疗计划，可能包含加入 各种自我戒酒团体，如社区内的互诚会或长期戒 酒组织。此外，建议参加由专业治疗师负责的戒酒群体。

# You can Do It 您可以做到

## OUTPATIENT DETOXES

### IF YOU CANNOT AFFORD AN INPATIENT PLAN OR ONE IS NOT AVAILABLE

若无法负担住院脱瘾治疗费用，或脱瘾机构无

法提供住院脱瘾治疗，则应采用门诊脱瘾治疗

Ideally, the individual should go in for an inpatient detox. In some countries where such facilities may not exist, an outpatient detox can also be attempted. The first step in such a detox is to make your resolution and set a date for when to start your detox. Here are some steps you can take in collaboration with your doctor for a successful outpatient detox:

理想情况下，酗酒者应住院进行脱瘾治疗。但在部分国家，可能没有提供这项服务的机构。因此，也可以采用门诊脱瘾治疗。这种治疗的第一步，就是要制定计划，并设定脱瘾治疗的开始日期。为了让门诊脱瘾治疗成功，您可以在医生的帮助下采取以下步骤：

- Make a resolution to stop drinking and set a date for your detox
  制定计划停止饮酒，并设定脱瘾治疗的 日期；

- Arrange for leave of 7 to 10 days from your work
  向单位请假 7 至 10 天；

- Consult with a doctor before hand and a trusted friend to assist you
  提前咨询医生，并向值得信赖的朋友寻求帮助；

- Have a stockpile of food and water

准备充足的食物与水；

- Remove all alcoholic drinks from home.
  丢掉家里所有的酒精饮料。

- Have someone stay with you during the detox.
  安排脱瘾期间的陪护人员；

- You can either decrease your drinking by 1/5 of your normal amount every day or have the doctor prescribe benzodiazepine medications for you with instructions on how to taper the dose.
  您可以每天按日常酒量的 1/5 减少饮酒，也可以服用医生开具的苯二氮平类药物，并按照说明逐渐减少服用量；

- Make sure the vitamin Thiamine 100 mg tablet and multivitamins are included.
  确保同时服用维生素类药物硫胺素 100 毫克片剂及复合维生素；

- If you develop excessive shaking or mental clouding or confusion, go to the emergency room to have the detox be completed under medical supervision.
  如果出现颤抖加剧、神志不清或意识模糊，请到急诊室就诊，在医院监护下完成脱瘾治疗；

- Stay well hydrated and well fed during the detox.
  脱瘾期间，要多饮水，补充营养，平衡膳食；

- Try to maintain routine activities such as going outdoors in your backyard for the sunshine and fresh air and doing some exercise
  努力保持日常活动，比如阳光充足、空气 清新时，就

# You can Do It 您可以做到

近进行户外活动及体育锻炼；

- Many individuals have been able to detox themselves. It happens all the time. Unsupervised detox however without consultation with a doctor and the presence of a trusted family member or friend is not recommended. Withdrawals can get complicated if the dependence is severe or if there are other medical problems.

  许多人都可以自行脱瘾，而且可以在任何时候　　实施。但不建议在没有监护、未咨询医生，及　　没有值得信赖的家庭成员陪护的情况下自行脱瘾。如果对酒精具有严重的依赖性，或存在其他的健康问题，停止饮酒会让病情复杂化。

- More expensive rehabilitation facilities cost a lot more but do not necessarily deliver better care than what you can obtain locally in a low- cost facility.

  更昂贵的脱瘾康复机构收费较高，但所　　提供的护理，也是与您从廉价机构所获得　　的护理无法相比的；

- The most important part of recovery is your sincerity and motivation to quit alcohol use and for making your life better.

  康复的关键，在于您为戒酒及让生活更美好所付出的真诚与积极；

- Fancy buildings and glitzy advertisements about treatment centers will not provide you success if you are yourself not fully committed to your recovery. It can be done and you can do it.

  如果没有对自己康复的全情投入，治疗　　中心奇特的建筑与炫目的广告，是不会让　　您脱瘾成功的。脱瘾是可以实现的，您可以做到。

- You can change your life around for the better.
  为了让自己的生活更好，您可以做出改变；

- Simple recommendations are sometimes the most effective tools in your arsenal. This includes going to groups, keeping busy and removing alcoholic beverages from the environment.
  在您可以选择的方法中，简单的建议有时就是最有效的手段，包括参加戒酒团体，让自己忙碌，并扔掉身边的酒精饮料。

## **COMBINATION** OF ALCOHOL WITH OTHER SEDATING MEDICATIONS **IS A DEADLY MIX**

## 酒精与其他镇静类药物**混用会致命**

When alcohol is mixed with other sedating medications, the combination can be lethal. Some of the recent celebrity deaths were due to a combination of a benzodiazepine, an opiate and alcohol.

酒精与其他镇静类药物混用会致命。最近，有社会名流就因混用具有麻醉作用的苯二氮平类药物与酒精而致死。

Alcohol alone in overdose can kill. Opiates such as heroin and Barbiturates alone can also kill in overdose. Benzodiazepines alone are usually not lethal in overdose but when combined with alcohol, they can be lethal. The combination can lead to a fatal suppression of the respiratory center. This means the person stops breathing and dies.

单独的饮酒过量可以致命；单独服用诸如吗啡及巴比妥类药物过量也可以致命。单独服用苯二氮平类药物过量通常不会致命，但当其与酒精混用时，就会致命。二者混用可以导致致命的呼吸系统抑制。这意味着服用者停止呼吸而亡。

Sedating medications should therefore never be combined with alcohol. If you are taking any such medications, do not drink alcohol.

因此，永远不要混用酒精与镇静类药物。如果您正在服用此类药物，就不要饮酒。

## INSURANCE FOR DETOX IS AVAILABLE UNDER THE AFFORDABLE HEALTHCARE ACT

按照《可负担医保法案》为脱瘾治疗投保是可行 的

Under the Obama care Affordable Health Care Act, coverage for inpatient detox and outpatient rehabilitation is guaranteed. Under a separate Mental Health Parity Act, equal coverage has been guaranteed for treatment mental health issues including alcohol and substance abuse problems. The treatment facility where you can get treatment commonly offers to help you get this insurance coverage for you if you do not have it. You're encouraged to check your local pages or the Internet for local treatment facilities. You can call them to see what kind of help they can offer in getting insurance paperwork completed for you.

按照奥巴马政府颁布的《可负担医保法案》，住 院脱瘾治疗与门诊脱瘾康复的费用都是得到保障  的。按照单独的《心理健康平权法案》，对于包  括酒精及物质滥用问题在内的心理健康问题的治  疗费用，也是得到同等保障的。通常，您接受治 疗的机构，会帮助您在没有获得这种保险的前提 下，成功投保。鼓励您查阅当地黄页，或登录互  联网查找当地治疗机构。您可以致电他们，了解  在完成投保方面，可以提供的帮助。

# You can Do It 您可以做到

## DISTRACT YOURSELF WHEN AN URGE ARISES.

酒瘾发作时，让自己转移注意力

If you have an urge or craving for alcohol, you can take some of the following steps. You can take a tablet of Antabuse or Calcium Carbimide if to put a barrier of unpleasant side effects if you drink. You can also distract yourself by listening to music, doing some exercise or by calling your sponsor or friend that knows you are in recovery. You can make it a game like riding a wave.

如果您有饮酒的冲动，或酒瘾发作，可以采取以下一些步骤：服用一片安塔布斯或氰胺钙，让自己在可能饮酒时出现令人不适的副作用，以此防止饮酒；还可以转移注意力，听听音乐、做一些运动，或同支持自己的人或朋友通电话，让他们知道您正处于康复之中。您可以把这当作一场与酒瘾的竞逐，就像冲浪。

When a craving arises, view it as an ocean wave. Bring your attention to the present moment and use your present moment awareness like a surf board. Staying in the present moment, you can be aware and stay above the urge. You will be surfing the urge and see the various thoughts and images flit through your mindscape but you choose to stay here in the moment. The more you do it, the more confident you will become in being able to resist the temptation. You have to tell yourself in the present moment that you are safe and will be safe if you don't give in. Also fill your time with other activities where you can be in the present moment with such as conversation with a friend or some work that interests you. If you repeatedly conquer the cravings, they will soon dissipate.

酒瘾发作时，将它视为一波海浪。让您的注意力停留在此刻，并把此刻的自我意识，当作一块冲浪板。让意识就此停驻，您会保持清醒，并战胜这种冲动。您能够驾驭这种冲动，正视出现在头脑中的各种想法和场景，只要您选择让意识就此停驻。越是这样，您越有信心拒绝诱惑。此刻，您必须告诫自己的是，自己是安全的，而且，如果不向这种冲动妥协，就可以保持安全。此外，利用眼前的时间让自己参与能够参与的其他活动，比如与朋友交谈，或做一些自己感兴趣的工作。如果您多次战胜这种冲动，不久，它们就会消失了。

# You can Do It 您可以做到

## ENGAGE IN MEDITATION OR QUIET TIME FOR 15 TO 20 MINUTES DAILY.

坚持药物治疗，或每天安排 15 至 20 分钟的安静
时间

Once a day, schedule about 15 to 20 minutes for yourself. Make it a regular scheduled activity and don't let other events intrude. Find a comfortable posture in a natural setting and let yourself relax by focussing on the natural rise and fall of your breath. Do not resist any thoughts that come and just bring your attention back to your breath. Not resisting any thoughts and not giving them energy allows the mind to come to a gradual standstill. Let whatever happens with the mind happen. If some images come or thoughts come, observe them and let them drift away. Like a spinning wheel that does not get the new energy of attention, the mind will begin to settle. Just enjoy the quiet time. You don't have to call it meditation but just call it quiet time. At the end of this exercise, visualize your goals for the day and your life. Visualize some mini goals and visualize them as already attained. Just do the exercise and leave it at that. Good things will begin to happen in your life. The moments of seeming nothingness are not wasted moments. These moments are moments of great potential for healing and achievement.

每天为自己安排一次约 15 至 20 分钟的安静时间。让它成为一种规律，不要因其他事情而中断。找到一种舒服而自然的姿势，将注意力集中到呼吸的自然节奏上，让自己放松。不要抗拒产生的任何想法，只要将自己的注意力带回到呼吸上即可。不要抗拒任何想法，也不要专注于它，让大脑逐渐停止思考即可。顺其自然。如果一些场景或想法出现了，正视它们，并让它们逐渐消失。如同旋转的车轮得不到能量的补充，大脑就会平静下来。而您，只要享受这安静时刻即可。您不必把这称为冥想，称之为安静时间即可。练习结束时，把你对这一天及人生的目

标具体化。把一些小目标具体化，就如同已经实现。进行这种练习，并坚持不断，您的生活将出现可喜的变化。这些安静时间看似无关致要，但都不是对生命的浪费。它们是可能治愈，并让您实现成功的伟大时刻。

To repeat, at the end of the quiet period, visualize the goals for about 5 minutes that you want for that day. Furthermore, imagine them to have already been achieved. Then when these goals and sub goals that you visualized become manifest, consider it to be par for the course. Let this make you stronger in your resolution to better your life and achieve your other goals.

要在安静时间结束时，用大约 5 分钟的时间，将您希望在当天完成的目标重新具体化。此外，想象它们已经实现了。随后，当您所具体化的这些目标及其子目标变为现实时，把它看作这种练习的标准。让这种练习使您在脱瘾治疗中更加强大，生活更加美好，并实现其他的目标。

I want to give credit for this method to two sources. One is the exercise of Transcendental Meditation. The other is the author and entrepreneur Trevor Blake. He advocates this in his wonderful book, Three Little Steps. I highly recommend this book. The three simple steps are

出于两种原因，我想赞美这种方法。原因之一，在于这可以锻炼冥思静坐；另一个原因则是作家兼企业家特雷弗·布雷克。在自己的佳作-- 《小小的三步》一书中，布雷克对这种方法进行了倡导。我极力向您推荐本书。书中所说的三步包括：

1. A positive mentality unyielding to doubt or negativity.
   面对怀疑或否定，抱有积极的心态；

2. A daily period of quiet time for 20 minutes in a natural,

quiet, peaceful setting.

在自然、宁静及平和的环境中，每天冥思静坐 20 分钟。

3. Visualization of positive goals you want to achieve and expecting them to be achieved in the depths of your heart with total conviction.
So schedule 15 to 20 minutes out of every day for yourself.. It is a simple technique but will be one of the most important tools in your arsenal.

具体化您想要实现的积极目标，并坚定而由衷地期待它们得以实现。因此，每天抽出 15 至 20 分钟冥思静坐。这是个简单的技巧，但会成为可以选择的方案中，您最重要的手段之一。

## COGNITIVE BEHAVIORAL THERAPY (CBT)
认知行为疗法（CBT）

This is a remarkable therapy that has a great appeal due to it's rugged logic. In this therapy, the therapist helps you recognize the nature of your thoughts, unstated underlying assumptions which may be erroneous and how these distorted thoughts may be affecting your emotions and in turn your behaviors. It also examines steps that can be taken to correct the distortions.

这是一种重要的治疗方法，因为逻辑严密，而具有巨大的影响力。采用这种疗法，治疗师会帮助您对自己想法的本质、没有表达的潜在设想进行认识。这些想法和设想可能是错误的，扭曲的思想可能会影响您的情绪，并随之对行为造成影响。此外，这种疗法还可以让人审视修正扭曲思想的有效步骤。

When exposed to the light of examination, the drive and the force behind that drinking behavior is examined, the triggers for cravings are identified. Later you and your therapist can create exercise to recognize any distortions associated with the trigger and also on how to defuse the trigger.

治疗的过程，是对酗酒背后的动机与诱惑的审视，也是对引起酗酒冲动原因的识别。稍后，您与自己的治疗师可以构想练习，找出与酗酒冲动原因相关的任何异常思想，以及除去这些原因的方法。

# You can Do It 您可以做到

## LEARN TO SHED THE STIGMA OF ALCOHOLISM
学会摆脱因酗酒而致的耻辱感

At some point, one has to shed the stigma related to alcohol use disorders. Alcoholism is a disease, and it needs to be treated without stigmatizing the sufferer. The disease of alcoholism does not respect occupation, education, wealth or other indicators of status. It is an illness and just like any other illness can afflict anyone.

有时，酗酒者必须要摆脱与酒精使用障碍有关的 耻辱感。酗酒是一种病态，需要酗酒者在不感受到耻辱的前提下接受治疗。它与职位、受教育程度、财富或其他的身份象征无关。它是一种疾病，同任何其他疾病一样，会让人痛苦。

## TAKE IT ONE DAY AT A TIME

把握每一天

Remember that you can overcome any long term challenge if you take life one day at a time.

记住，您可以战胜任何长期的挑战，只要把握每一天。

Thinking of long term goals can seem daunting. If you however see your goals as being near term, the challenge is more manageable. You can only live your life in the now, so focus your efforts at keeping your stability in the now, for this moment, and for this day. Use the coping skills for managing your urges and anxieties and your days will spread into months and years of a happy and sober life for you and your family.

对长期目标的思索，这可能让人感到困难。但是，如果将其视为近期目标，就容易多了。活在当下，关注自己为保持目前、此刻以及今天生活稳定而付出的努力即可。运用冲动与焦虑的相应管理技巧，您的生活会长时间地保持快乐，让自己与家人拥有宁静的日子。

# You can Do It 您可以做到

## YOU WILL SEE IMPROVEMENT DAY BY DAY AFTER DETOX

### 脱瘾后，您会看到生活逐渐改善

You will notice your strength and physical stability improving day by day after the first week. The areas of skin where dandruff and dryness were present will begin to resolve. You will also notice your memory improving as well as your ability to focus and concentrate. Other welcome changes may center on an improved mood, and an increasing self-confidence within you. You will notice your irritability and anxiety begin to resolve. Some of this anxiety before was centered around the obtaining of the next drink and avoiding withdrawal. All the different organs affected by toxicity of alcohol begin to show an improvement. Even your liver will begin to regenerate with an improvement in your physical health. Relationships and libido also improve with continuing sobriety. You have all this to look forward to by overcoming and quitting alcohol.

脱瘾一周后，您会看到自己体能与健康的稳定改善。曾经干燥起皮的皮肤，开始富有光泽；记忆力开始恢复，注意力变得集中。其他令人欣喜的变化，可能主要出现在情绪改善方面，以及自信心的增长，及烦躁与焦虑开始得到改善。 以前的焦虑，主要因为再次地饮酒及不愿戒酒。所有受到酒精不良影响的不同身体器官，开始呈现出改善。甚至您的肝脏也会开始伴随健康状况的改善而再生。家庭关系及性的冲动也随着持续的戒酒而得到改善。所有这一切，都是您通过摆脱酗酒及戒酒会得到的。

# HOW ALCOHOLISM BE A BAIT AND SWITCH
## 酗酒如何成为一种诱饵与转折

When you take an alcoholic drink for the first time, you may experience an initial euphoria on low doses of alcohol. This euphoria however soon vanishes and leaves you in a state that is lower than where you began. You have a 15% chance of being in a special population that has a higher risk of becoming addicted. Repeated use leads to tolerance and the need for more alcohol to achieve the effect. Soon, there is no positive effect, and you are always in the pit that comes afterward. You in fact never come out of the pit and are soon drinking just to stay normal. Soon, no amount of alcohol works and on top of this, you have physical symptoms of withdrawal even while there is alcohol in your blood stream. This is the nightmare that alcohol perpetrates year after year on millions of people. The many complications related to alcoholism begin to cascade through your life. It may begin with a job loss, a divorce, a jail term for DUI, prison time for other charges and perhaps an early death due to disease or an accident. Not what you imagined with that first small drink.

初次饮酒时,您可能会经历最初少量饮酒后的愉悦。然而，这种感觉不久就消失了，留下的感觉比开始时更糟糕。您有 15% 的机会，成为具有较高成瘾风险的特殊人群中的一员。反复饮酒，导致为获得舒适感受，而对更大饮酒量的耐受与需求。不久，饮酒就不会为您带来积极的感受了，而您则在随后酗酒成瘾。事实上，您从未摆脱酒瘾，并很快让它成为了平常行为。稍后，相当的酒量就已经对您不起作用了。更要命的是，您出现了停止饮酒症状，即便还有酒精残留在您的血液中。年复一年，数百万人沉迷饮酒之中，这是一场噩梦。与酗酒相关的许多不良连锁反应开始不断出现在您生活中。开始可能是失业、离婚、因酒驾被拘留、由于其他指控获刑入狱，又或许因疾病或意外事故而提前离世。最初一小口所带来的影响，令人出乎意料。

How is that for bait and switch with a little drink that began with a warm, gentle euphoria.

这一小口，之所以成为诱饵与转折，发端于一次温暖、舒适的精神愉悦。

The person with alcohol problem has a false perception of his situation. Society and prior social conditioning predispose the trusting person to accept the lies about the benign nature of alcohol via the false advertisements.

存在酗酒问题的人，错误地看待自己的处境。社会与先前的社会条件作用，让容易轻信他人的人偏向于在虚假广告词的作用下，接受关于酒精本质上无害的谎言。

If one were to be fully aware of the problem, their desire for alcohol would be gone, and they would never touch it. We are tricked and deceived by the trendy and glitzy media ads, while the real dangers of alcohol remain deliberately hidden.

如果一个人能充分意识到这个问题，他们就不会有酗酒的愿望。不仅如此，还滴酒不沾。媒体广告语，时尚、炫目。它让我们受到戏弄与欺骗，与此同时，却把酒精真正的危险精心地隐藏起来。

## NALMEFENE IS SIMILAR TO NALTREXONE AND HAS BEEN FOUND TO BE EFFECTIVE FOR ALCOHOL PROBLEMS

### 纳美芬类似于纳曲酮的有效戒酒作用已被发现

Nalmefene is also a long-acting opiate antagonist like naltrexone and can be helpful in curbing the cravings and dysfunctional use of alcohol in a way similar to naltrexone. The advantage is that it has fewer side effects and is better tolerated.

纳美芬也是一种长效麻醉拮抗药，类似于纳曲酮。可以一种近似于纳曲酮的方式，帮助抑制酒瘾及滥饮。其优势在于对人体的副作用更少，耐受性更好。

Nalmefene is currently not available in the United States.

目前，美国境内不允许使用纳美芬。

# You can Do It 您可以做到

## CALCIUM CARBIMIDE TO STOP DRINKING
### 服用氰胺钙期间不能饮酒

This is a salt sold under the brand name Temposil and Abstem in the United States.

在美国，氰胺钙是一种出售的盐，品牌名称为 Temposil 和 Abstem。

It's mechanism of action is similar to Antabuse. It may be easier on the liver than Antabuse for some people. If you drink alcohol on top of this medication, you will experience reactions similar to when Antabuse is combined with alcohol. This is because the mechanism of action is similar. It too stops the breakdown of alcohol at the intermediate acetaldehyde level. Rising acetaldehyde levels will cause you to be nauseated, vomit or experience other distressful side effects. Knowing that you will experience the unpleasant effects if you drink, you are less likely to start drinking after taking calcium carbimide or Antabuse.

氰胺钙对人体的作用机理，近似于安塔布斯。对某些人而言，它比安塔布斯更易被肝脏吸收。如果在服用本药后饮酒，您的感受会同安塔布斯与饮酒混合时的反应相似。这是因为它们具有类似的作用机理。氰胺钙也可以使酒精中间代谢产物乙醛的降解受阻。乙醛水平在人体内的升高，会引起恶心、呕吐，或感受其他令人不适的副作用。懂得饮酒后会经历的不适，您在服用氰胺钙或安塔布斯后饮酒的可能性就会更小。

Calcium Carbimide and Antabuse should only be used in consultation with a doctor. They are not recommended if you are pregnant, diabetic or have heart disease.

氰胺钙和安塔布斯都只能遵医嘱服用。如果您是孕妇、糖尿病患者，或患有心脏病，不建议使用这两种药物。

# You can Do It 您可以做到

## HELP SHOULD BE PROVIDED FOR OTHER FAMILY MEMBERS AS WELL.

### 其他家庭成员也应该获得帮助

All the members of a family are affected, and they may have feelings about the problems caused by alcohol in their lives. Certain support groups such as Al-Anon do offer support to family members through the self-help group model. Sharing the trials and tribulations with other afflicted family members can help reduce the stigma, helplessness, and depression a family member may feel. They may take hope from each other. If a doctor recognizes that a family member is having significant problems with depression or other psychiatric disorder, help can be offered to the sick family member.

所有家庭成员无一例外地受到酗酒问题的影响。或许在他们的生活中，也有因此而引起的各种情绪。某些支持组织，如匿名戒酒者协会，就通过自助群体模式，为酗酒者的家庭成员提供帮助。与其他受到酗酒问题困扰家庭的成员分享痛苦与难过，这可以有助于使家庭成员可能感受到的耻辱感、无助感及压抑感减轻。如果医生发现家庭成员正在出现严重抑郁或其他心理问题，可以为患病家庭成员提供帮助。

Al Anon groups in your local area can be found at the following website.

http://www.al-anon.alateen.org/find-a-meeting

登陆以下网站，您可以找到所在地区的匿名戒酒者协会：

http://www.al-anon.alateen.org/find-a-meeting

If you are an alcoholic, you can share this information with your family member so that they can utilize this resource.

如果您是酗酒者，可以与自己的家人分享这些信息，便于他们利用这些资源。

# INVOLUNTARY TREATMENT CAN BE USED TO STOP DRINKING

## 可以用非自愿治疗方法戒酒

Most people don't know that a family member may be able to commit you involuntarily to a facility for treatment. The petitioner has to allege that there is a risk to the life of the individual, or a family member if treatment is not provided to the individual. If you the alcoholic do not contest, the judge will allow the commitment. If you try to contest this, it becomes a little more difficult but may still happen. After the inpatient detox, a judge can order outpatient treatment as well. Legislation may vary in different areas. You should search for the laws in your local area regarding commitment for treatment of alcohol and substance abuse disorders.

绝大多数人认为，家庭成员不会让酗酒者进入机构进行

非自愿戒酒治疗。这种疗法的支持者们一定会辩称，如果不进行治疗，酗酒者会存在生命危险。如果作为酗酒者，您对此不置可否，法庭会同意对您采取这种戒酒方法；如果您设法为此争辩，那么，对您实施该疗法就会有难度，但还是有发生的可能。强制脱瘾后，法庭也会下令您接受门诊治疗。不同地区，相关规定不尽相同。您应该查阅所在地与酒精及物质滥用问题相关的法律规定。

## HUMILITY AND ALCOHOLICS ANONYMOUS
谦逊与匿名酗酒互助会

One of the key drivers of alcoholism and substance abuse is the sense of self-importance and the feeling that one can outsmart the addiction.

酒精与物质滥用的关键诱因之一，在于人的自负感，以及认为自己能够想办法战胜它而不上瘾。

When one makes a sincere confession of one's failings, one begins for the first time an affair with honesty. This honesty and humility allows one to look past the illusion of control that interferes with getting a true appreciation of the problem.

真正承认失败，就是诚实对事的开始。这种诚实与谦逊，可以使人放弃对自我控制能力的幻想，不让它对真实地看待问题形成干扰。

The road to recovery in meetings of the Alcoholic Anonymous also begins with this state of humility. AA (Alcoholic Anonymous) starts by accepting the powerlessness over alcohol. This seems like it is disempowering, but it is the most empowering thing because it is the truth. It empowers them to ally themselves with their higher natures, their higher powers and be single minded in the efforts towards recovery instead of keeping pretenses about being able to control the problem on their own. If they could have controlled it on their own, they already would have and would not be in a world of hurt they find themselves in. The AA prayer is very thoughtful and reminds us to not be inactive but to do what we can. It is as follows:

"God grant me the serenity to accept the things I cannot change; courage to change the things I can and wisdom to know the difference,"

匿名戒酒互助会的康复之路，也始于这种谦逊。互诚会（匿名戒酒互助会）认可酗酒者对于酒精的无法抗拒，以此开始为酗酒者提供帮助。这看似对酗酒的无能为力，但却是最强大的帮助，因为这是事实。互诚会让酗酒者有能力秉承自己更本真的天性、更强大的力量，一心一意地为脱瘾康复而努力，而不过分夸大依靠自身对问题进行控制的能力。如果可以依靠自己控制饮酒量，酗酒者已经而且也不会发现自己身处伤害之中了。如下所示的互诚会祈祷语，富有深意，能提醒我们积极地做力所能及的事：

"上帝赐予我们宁静，接受无法改变的一切；鼓励我们改变能够改变的一切，并清醒认识其中的差异。"

Overcoming Alcohol 摆脱酗酒

# FINDING SOURCES FOR HELP

## 找到资源，寻求帮助

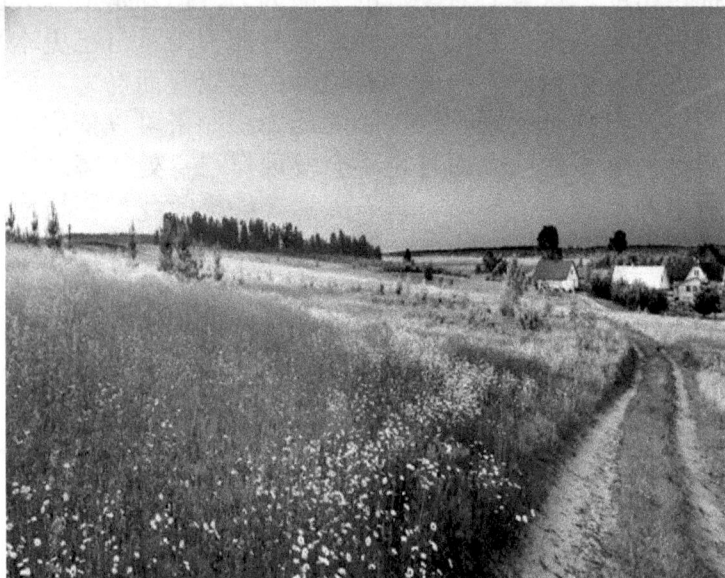

# You can Do It 您可以做到

## A WEBSITE FOR AA MEETINGS

互诚会网站

The below website can find you a local AA meeting in the United States, Canada and some other countries as well.

登录以下网站，您可以找到美国、加拿大及其他国家的当地互诚会。

It is at http://www.aa.org/

网址是：http://www.aa.org/

# Overcoming Alcohol 摆脱酗酒

## A REFERRAL HOTLINE FOR DETOX CENTERS

脱瘾中心推荐热线电话

This line is manned 24/7 and can provide you a referral to a detox center near you. Their toll free number is Tel 1-877-998-5411

该热线提供每周 7 天、每天 24 小时的人工接听服务，为 您推荐附近的脱瘾中心。他们的免费电话是：

电话：1-877-998-5411

## You can Do It 您可以做到

## A WEBSITE TO FIND TREATMENT CENTERS

可以找到治疗中心的网站

The below website can help you locate some local treatment centers

https://addictiontosobriety.com/alcohol-rehab/?utm_source=bing&utm_campaign=b6&utm_medium=c&utm_content=0436A00001

以下网站可以帮助您确定当地治疗中心的所在位置:

https://addictiontosobriety.com/alcohol-

rehab/?utm_source=bing&utm_campaign=b6&utm_mediu

m=c&utm_content=0436A00001

# Overcoming Alcohol 摆脱酗酒

## FOR DEVOUT CHRISTIANS: CELEBRATE RECOVERY GROUPS

适用于虔诚基督教徒的脱瘾机构：欢庆痊愈组织

This is a Christian based group started by Pastor Christopher Warren of Saddleback Church in Phoenix. He had earlier written a best-selling book, The Purpose Driven Life. There is an emphasis on Bible backed principles. There is an emphasis on addressing past "hurts, hang-ups and habits."

这是一个以基督教徒为主的组织，由菲尼克斯赛德贝克教堂牧师克里斯托弗·华伦发起。较早前，华伦撰写了一本畅销书《目标驱动生活》，强调圣经所支持的信念，并着重解决过去的"伤痛、烦恼与习惯"。

This means that the person is allowed to bring up and address any past traumas, and allowed to examine behaviors resultant from this. The habitual ways of dealing with the anxieties may be functional or dysfunctional. The alcohol habit is seen as a dysfunctional habit, and spiritual strength and insight are used to break the habit. This is done in the context of spiritual and emotional support from the group.

这意味着个体得以说出并解决过去的任何心理创伤，审视由此而导致的各种自身行为。应对焦虑的习惯方式，可能是正常的，也可能是异常的。酗酒被看作是异常习惯，而常常用以破除它的是个体内心的强大及深刻认识。在该组织所提供的精神及情感支持下，酗酒习惯能够得以破除。

Their website is celebraterecovery.com

组织网址是：celebraterecovery.com

It can be a great resource for those that have strong religious faith and are trying to quit alcohol.

对于那些具有强烈宗教信仰，正努力戒酒的人而言，这

个机构作用显著。

# Overcoming Alcohol 摆脱酗酒

## TREATMENT BY SECULAR SELF-HELP GROUPS
接受长期自助戒酒组织的治疗

Some individuals may prefer not to have religious beliefs imposed on them by attending the 12 step AA groups. These are called secular self-help groups.

有些人可能更不喜欢因参与 12 步戒酒疗法互诚会，而让自己信仰宗教。那么，您可以参与长期自助戒酒组织。

In these groups, there is a greater emphasis on looking at internal factors unique to the individual that predispose to addiction. The individual is encouraged to take whatever steps are under their control to lessen their risk. The responsibility for one's recovery is placed entirely on the person himself. He or she is empowered to believe that he can do this by understanding the addictive forces and making active plans to defeat such triggers. In some ways, the AA and NonAA secular groups have some similarities. In AA, there is a greater emphasis on spirituality, humility and asking for help while the person does the things he or she can. In Secular Groups, there is a greater emphasis on the ability of an individual to defeat the forces of addiction through an understanding of the disease process and making a sincere desire to quit alcohol.

这些组织更注重看到让个体偏向于成瘾的特定内因，这种内因因人而异。个体受到鼓励而采取的任何减少自己风险的步骤，都受到组织的主导。个体康复的责任，完全由自己承担。组织赋予他或她力量，让他们相信自己能够借助对成瘾力的理解，以及制定战胜诱惑的积极计划，完成脱瘾。就某些方面而言，互诚会与非互诚会长期自助戒酒组织有着诸多的相似之处。互诚会更注重精神意识、谦逊的品格，以及在个体从事力所能及之事时所寻求的帮助。长期自助戒酒组织则更注重个体通过对病程的理解，以及树立戒酒的真正愿望，而战胜成瘾力的能力。

Similar to AA, attendance of regular groups is still recommended for consolidating recovery.

仍然推荐您参与与互诚会相似的常规戒酒组织，对康复进行巩固。

Some of these are as follows.

其中一些常规戒酒组织如下：

WOMEN FOR SOBRIETY (WFS) GROUPS: The founder Jean Kirkpatrick recognized that the issues of woman alcoholics are different. This is true as there is a greater prevalence of depression and other emotional issues in many women that are alcoholic. Treatment of the depression can improve the prognosis significantly for these women. The women are encouraged to work on their self-esteem and get help for depression as needed.

女性戒酒组织：创始人简·科克派翠克认为，女性酗酒与男性不同。这是事实，女性因酗酒而出现抑郁和其他情绪问题的人更多。对抑郁的治疗，可以极大地改善这些女性的预后状况。该组织鼓励女性自尊，并在需要时，为治疗抑郁而获取帮助。

More information can be found at womenforsobriety.org

更多信息，可登陆**网站** womenforsobriety.org 获取。

SMART RECOVERY GROUPS: In this groups of recovering alcoholics, there is a greater emphasis on cognitive behavior therapy (CBT). The group members are also encouraged to empower themselves to believe they can overcome their illness. They are encouraged to make every effort towards that end. Their website is smartrecovery.org

斯玛特康复组织：该组织更注重认知行为疗法。组织成员都受到鼓励，相信自己能战胜疾病，并尽一切努力战胜疾病。组织的网站是：smartrecovery.org

SECULAR ORGANIZATION FOR SOBRIETY (SOS) is a similar organization with similar beliefs. Staying sober is the prime focus and directive for group members. Many individuals find this approach helpful. Their website is sossobriety.org

长期戒酒组织（SOS）是一个具有类似信仰的类似组织。适度饮酒，并为组织成员提供指导，是组织的首要关注点。许多人发现这种方法非常有效。他们的网站是 sossobriety.org

LIFERING SECULAR RECOVERY: This organization states it's emphasis to be the following three goals: sobriety, secularity, and self-help. Their website is as follows: http://lifering.org/

终身康复组织：该组织表示将以下三个目标作为自己的关注点：戒酒、平常心与自我帮助。他们的网站如下：http://lifering.org/

# You can Do It 您可以做到

## EPILOGUE
## 结语

I hope this book gave you some ideas for recovery from alcohol. You can use this knowledge now to talk to your doctor. The doctor can guide you about detox and subsequent recovery options. As you know now, there are many options. If you are well yourself, but know someone who is struggling with alcohol, you can share the knowledge that recovery is possible. Sometimes, a solitary word of support and a single ray of hope can guide a person out of their darkness. Be supportive of those that suffer because alcoholism is a disease and not a sign of moral weakness. There should therefore be no shame or stigma about alcoholism. You would not be ashamed of having heart disease or diabetes if the disease ran in your family and your genes put you at risk for it. Alcoholism is no different. Up to 50 percent of the risk for alcoholism is inherited. The enlightened approach is to accept the disease of alcoholism when it exists and modify the other 50 percent that is under your control. A part of this effort should be to avoid exposure to alcohol. With knowledge you gained from this simple book, you can overcome alcohol. Just get detoxed under medical supervision, and make a plan to keep on the path of sobriety. It is that simple. May The Higher Power Aid Your Efforts. God Speed!

TSG

希望本书能为您的戒酒康复，提供一些思路。现在，您可以运用这些知识，与医生进行探讨。让他在脱瘾及后续的康复方案选择中，对您进行引导。正如您所知，目前的脱瘾治疗方法多种多样。如果您康复了，也认识正在为戒酒而抗争的其他人，那就告诉他脱瘾康复是可以实现的。有时，一句支持的话语和一缕希望的光芒，可以引导人走出困境。为那些承受酗酒之痛的人提供帮助，因为酗酒是一种病，不是道德缺陷的标志。因此，不必为酗酒感到羞耻或耻辱。如果您的家族有心脏病或糖尿病史，而基因将您置于这种病的风险之中，您不会为此感到羞耻或耻辱。酗酒就与此类似。遗传带来的酗酒风险高达50%。开明的做法，是在嗜酒成瘾后，接受这种病的存在，并改变自己可以控制的其余 50%风险。这种努力就包含不饮酒。借助从这本简单易懂的书中所获得的知识，您可以摆脱酗酒。要在医院监督下脱瘾，并制定计划，坚持戒酒。就这么简单。上帝会帮助您。祝您成功！

TSG

You can Do It 您可以做到

## OTHER BOOKS BY THE AUTHOR

本书作者的其他著作

OVERCOMING ANXIETY

摆脱焦虑

HTTPS://WWW.AMAZON.COM/OVERCOMING-

ANXIETY-TIRATH-GILL-MD-

EBOOK/DP/B00L9NCKM8/REF=SR_1_2?IE=UTF8&QID=1480
015447&SR=82&KEYWORDS=TIRATH+S+GILL

## OVERCOMING SCHIZOPHRENIA

摆脱精神分裂症

HTTPS://www.amazon.com/Schizophrenia-Guide-Patients-Families-Clinicians/dp/0989664945/ref=sr_1_3?ie=UTF8&qid=1480015563&sr=8-3&keywords=Tirath+S+Gill

### DELIVERED FROM ADHD

原发性注意力不集中症

HTTPS://www.amazon.com/Delivered-ADHD-Overcoming-Children-Adults/dp/1463663404/ref=sr_1_fkmr0_2?ie=UTF8&qid=1480016395&sr=8-2-fkmr0&keywords=delivered+from+adhd+tirith

### USMLE Step 1 Short Summaries: A Ladder for Success

美国执业医师考试第 1 步 简要综述：成功的阶梯

HTTPS://www.amazon.com/USMLE-Step-Short-Summaries-Success/dp/0989664988/ref=sr_1_4?ie=UTF8&qid=1480015883&sr=8-4&keywords=TIRATH+S+GILL+MD

## You can Do It 您可以做到

## HANDBOOK OF EMERGENCY PSYCHIATRY,

精神疾病急救指南

HTTPS://www.amazon.com/Handbook-Emergency-    Psychiatry-Hani-   Khouzam/dp/0323040888/ref=sr_1_6?ie=UTF8&qid=1480 016641&sr=8-6&keywords=TIRATH+GILL

## HOW TO ACHIEVE YOUR GOALS: LEADERSHIP LESSONS FROM ALEXANDER THE GREAT

https://www.amazon.com/How-Achieve-Your-Goals-Leadership/dp/0989664902/ref=sr_1_1?ie=UTF8&qid=148 1186087&sr=8-1&keywords=tirath+s+gill+alexander

www.ingramcontent.com/pod-product-compliance
Lightning Source LLC
Chambersburg PA
CBHW060456280326
41933CB00014B/2768